Surfing the

blues

Dedicated to

George, Natalie and Tanya,
Infant of Prague,
Sacred Heart

With love

Surfing the
blues

A guide to
understanding and
coping with mood
disorders, panic
attack and manic-
depressive illness

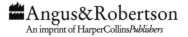
Angus&Robertson
An imprint of HarperCollins*Publishers*

Angus & Robertson
An imprint of HarperCollins*Publishers*, (Australia)

First published in Australia in 1996
by HarperCollins*Publishers* Pty Limited
ACN 009 913 517
A member of the HarperCollins*Publishers* (Australia) Pty Limited Group

HarperCollins*Publishers*
25 Ryde Road, Pymble, Sydney NSW 2073, Australia
31 View Road, Glenfield, Auckland 10, New Zealand
77–85 Fulham Palace Road, London W6 8JB, United Kingdom
Hazelton Lanes, 55 Avenue Road, Suite 2900, Toronto, Ontario, M5R 3L2
and 1995 Markham Road, Scarborough, Ontario M1B 5M8, Canada
10 East 53rd Street, New York NY 10032, USA

The National Library of Australia Cataloguing-in-Publication data:

Rzecki, Catherine.
  Surfing the blues : a guide to understanding and coping
  with mood disorders.

  ISBN 0 207 18866 1.

  1. Rzecki, Catherine – Mental health. 2. Panic attacks –
  Popular works. 3. Manic-depressive psychoses – Popular
  works. 4. Depression, Mental – Popular works. I. Title.

616.895

Designed by Rosemarie Franzoni
Cover design by Rosemarie Franzoni
Cover photograph *Untitled 1978* by Bill Henson
Typeset in Sabon by J&M Typesetting
Printed in Australia by Griffin Paperbacks

9 8 7 6 5 4 3 2 1
99 98 97 96

Our thanks go to those who have given us permission to reproduce
copyright material in this book. Particular sources of print material
are acknowledged in the text. Every effort has been made to contact
the copyright holders of print material, and the publisher welcomes
communication from any copyright holder from whom permission
was inadvertently not gained.

Acknowledgments

I wish to express my deep gratitude to those who took the time to respond to my questionnaire. The sharing of their experiences has added a depth to this book which would not otherwise have been possible. All names have been withheld and, where requested, identities disguised for the sake of confidentiality.

I am also deeply grateful to Association of Relatives and Friends of the Emotionally and Mentally Ill (ARAFEMI) Victoria and, in particular, Judith Player, who not only offered encouragement and support, but distributed the questionnaires and forwarded the responses on to me.

My thanks also go to Ashim Marfatia, Pharmacist, and Peter Murdoch, School Principal, who provided me with letters of reference, and to the small band of people who saved the day with their technical computer expertise when technology failed me: Ross Schnioffsky, Noel Stewart, Larry Wishart and John Grieve.

To those who provided research material and/or general support I also offer my most sincere thanks. They include Professor Graham D. Burrows, Austin Hospital, Heidelberg; Clinical Associate Professor Channa P. Wijesinghe, Footscray Psychiatric Hospital; Associate Professor Patrick McGorry, Royal Park Hospital, Parkville, and Kerryn Pennell of the Early Psychosis Prevention and Intervention Centre, Parkville; Associate Professor Philip Mitchell of The Prince Henry Hospital, Little Bay; Ashim Marfatia, Pharmacist, Williamstown; Andrew Fuller, Psychologist, Austin Hospital, Heidelberg; Dr Meg Smith OAM, University of Western Sydney and Depressive and Manic Depressive Association of NSW; Gwenda Cannard, Director of Tranquilliser Recovery and New Existence Inc. (TRANX) Melbourne for the information relating to tranquillisers and drug dependency; Robyn Sanderson of MANDA Newcastle Organisation; Geoff Rowcroft of Tobin Bros Melbourne; Glenda Johnston of the Directorate of School Education, Melbourne; Megan McQueenie of the Australian National Association for Mental Health; Pat Daniels of Canberra Manic-

Depressive Support Group; Even Keel Manic-Depressive Support Association Inc. WA; the Mental Health Association of the Northern Territory; Scott McBernie, Health & Community Services, Victoria; Leonie Manns of Mental Health Co-ordinating Council, Sydney; ARAFEMI Victoria for permission to reprint sections of certain articles from ARAFEMI Newsletters; Peter Curran and Marcia Christensen for assistance in procuring certain reference material; Mikela Sanderson for her Coping Strategies for Depression.

I am also deeply grateful to those members of the medical profession who gave most generously of their time to read my manuscript and provide their professional critiques and support, and I similarly appreciate the time spent by Sherryl Clark, Sharon Welgus and Laurel Hynes in reading and evaluating the manuscript in its early stages.

Without the generosity and assistance of all these people, this book would never have seen the light of day.

Lastly, but most importantly, I thank my family, George, Natalie and Tanya, for their support and encouragement, and for the forbearance shown at those times when my computer seemed more important than preparing dinner or tackling the ironing. Without their patience and support, this book would never have eventuated.

Foreword

I first met Catherine Rzecki in 1978 when I started taking lessons in painting and sketching from her mother-in-law Aleksandra. I spent many enjoyable hours with Aleksandra in her studio where she taught aspiring artists how to produce quality work. Catherine, too, spent many hours working in that studio, eventually selling a lot of her works. In time, as her daughters Natalie and Tanya grew older, they too learned from their grandmother.

I soon became the family physician and, in that capacity, I had the opportunity of getting to know the whole family well.

I watched Natalie and Tanya grow from young children, maturing into young women, nurtured in the close family unit that was so important to Catherine who, although she worked outside the home and spent many hours painting, always put the family first – to the extent that she eventually decided to abandon her painting as a hobby so that she could devote more time to the needs of her family.

The state of her health had fluctuated over the years, with the symptoms of stress-related disorders arising from time to time. A number of problems come to mind, including the removal of a cancerous melanoma early in 1987. But of course no one could have expected the illness that struck her later in 1987 – manic-depressive illness.

I remember when she first approached me in 1988, after having undergone extensive hypnotherapy. She was taking tranquillisers at the time, and I had to encourage her to gradually wean herself off them. I saw her a number of times, endeavouring to find a cause for the anxiety that was troubling her, but with little success. Eventually I referred her to a psychiatrist for help.

For a time the illness wreaked havoc on Catherine and her family. She struggled to comprehend and cope with it, her young daughters tried to come to terms with their mother's withdrawn behaviour which was so totally unexpected and difficult to understand, and her husband George tried to understand this strange new person who was his wife. For a time the family was completely devastated, with George and Catherine splitting up and the family home being put on the market.

Eventually, however, after a lot of upheaval, battles between all the family members and many inward struggles and soul-searching, each person found his or her own way of dealing with the problem, adopting strategies of coping.

Catherine has continued to improve and, although she still has frequent mood swings, those swings are not so severe and are of shorter duration.

She has proved her determination and her ability to cope with adversity by thoroughly researching the illness with which she has been afflicted, and has combined her research with her own personal experience to produce this book, hoping that it will be of great benefit to other sufferers and their families.

Dr S. Selvendra

Contents

Introduction

What are mood disorders?

This is a book about mood changes, fear, isolation and loneliness, but above all it is about courage, determination and hope in the face of overwhelming odds.

We have all experienced sudden, inexplicable changes in our mood – those days when we want to just curl up in bed and shut out the world, or we are bubbling over with energy and enthusiasm. Even though there might be no apparent reason for these shifts in mood, we do not usually pay them too much attention, because we know that they come and go, and they do not impinge on our lives to any great extent.

In some people, however, these shifts in mood are so exaggerated, both in intensity and duration, that they interfere dramatically with everyday living. They are unrelated to events such as traumatic loss or exhilarating experience, and depart so significantly from what we consider to be normal variations in mood, that they constitute a disorder or illness.

Unfortunately, most people have great difficulty understanding mood disorders. They see sufferers merely as moody, unstable, and unwilling to 'pull themselves together', and this attitude is exacerbated by an inability or unwillingness to discuss the illness because of the stigma attached to it or because they do not yet understand what is happening to them. I doubt that many people unacquainted with mental illness would consider that mood disorders constitute a very real physical pain as well as an exquisite mental anguish, neither of which can be controlled without medication. It seems sad, in this enlightened age where the media devotes so much time to such a wide range of informative topics, that over the years so little time has been devoted to mental illness.

Mood disorders have always been with us. They are considered to be the 'common cold' of major psychiatric illnesses, tending to concentrate in families, and affecting about one person in every hundred in Australia.

Written description of mood disorders dates back to Pharaonic Egypt, but the credit for the detailed description of this disorder and its separation from schizophrenia is given to the German psychiatrist, Emil Kraepelin. Through his work with the mentally ill at the end of the nineteenth century, he laid the foundations for modern psychiatry by meticulously describing the symptoms of mental illness, chronicling case histories and emphasising the *course of illness* as a major distinction between manic-depressive illness and the illness we now know as schizophrenia.

In the nineteenth century, those suffering from mental illness would have been confined to an asylum, to be ignored by the general population, but today, once manic-depressive illness is diagnosed and treated, the sufferer can look forward to leading a relatively normal life. This is due to the discovery in the 1950s of antimanic and antidepressant medications, the more recent development of reliable diagnostic systems, and the new medications that are frequently coming onto the market.

I hope that, by sharing my own and others' knowledge and experiences, other sufferers will gain a better understanding and acceptance of this illness and the often associated disorders of anxiety and agoraphobia, and that they, their family and friends, may be given a measure of comfort and hope for the future.

I hope, too, that the others who read this book, whether out of interest in health issues generally, or to gain further insight into how we can overcome the obstacles we so often find in our path during this lifetime, will discover that it can be rewarding and enriching to enter into the lives of other people. I am sure that this book will demonstrate that people suffering from a particular illness are 'normal', and just battling to come to terms with it and return to a former state of well-being.

Why this book?

There is nothing special that equips me to write this book other than the fact that I have been affected by anxiety, then agoraphobia and manic-depressive illness, since 1987. These disorders are really quite ordinary, but their effects are often anything but ordinary and need to be talked about more freely than they often are.

At age forty-two, when I experienced the first of this particular series of anxiety attacks, I was as much at peace with myself and life in general as most people are, considering life's usual ups and downs. I had certainly had my fair share of these, coming as I did from a family where anxiety or nervous disorders had become accepted as something we all had to learn to come to terms with, willingly or otherwise.

I originally decided to document my illness specifically for my family. When I was too ill to understand what it was doing to them, my husband George, and daughters Natalie and Tanya, endured an enormous emotional upheaval, not fully understanding what was happening to me, aware only that it was very quickly destroying all our lives. They had their responsibilities at work and school whilst at the same time coping with the bewilderment, embarrassment and frustration brought about by this disruptive illness. My parents, brother and sisters, on the other hand, all live interstate and have had little idea of what this illness is and how it has affected me. I hoped, by recording my knowledge and experiences, to help all of them become more familiar with the illness, how it has affected me, and how it has affected all our relationships.

But, somewhere along the way, I remembered the early days in my illness when I felt so desperately alone, chained to the stigma of an illness I could not accept and which those around me denied, thinking I was going through menopause. I leaned heavily on my psychiatrist for support, but at times even he was not enough. I needed to talk with someone who had experienced what I was experiencing, in order to fully understand and accept what was happening to me. But there was no one. What's more, for the first two years I could not find one book that recorded others' experiences. I scoured library and bookshop shelves and found a proliferation of books on depression, but in each one the author stated firmly that manic-depressive illness was not covered because it was a mental illness, different from regular depression, and must be treated separately. Nevertheless, I read these books, dozens of them, hoping to find even a few words I could relate to, although I recognised instinctively that I was suffering from something vastly different from what they described.

Two years later I finally did find a book dealing purely with manic-depressive illness. There were no words to describe my relief. The authors had included the personal accounts of a number of ordinary people like myself, and I discovered that their bizarre feelings and experiences were exactly the same as mine. I hugged the book to my chest, breathing a prayer of thanks. At last I knew I was not alone, and it no longer mattered that friends and family could not believe or accept that I was indeed suffering from a mental illness over which I had no control. I knew, I believed, and finally I was able to accept my illness for what it was – as real as any other such as diabetes. At last I felt real hope for the future. No matter how much I had to suffer, I would now be able to find the patience to endure it, to become well again as others had done before me.

These thoughts led me to the decision that I must write a more extensive book, which I would make available to other people suffering from this illness, and their families, in the hope that I might bring a little understanding, acceptance and hope into their lives.

First episodes of any of these disorders can be very scary, and so I have deliberately not held back in describing the effects I encountered, in order that others will have something to relate to when faced with a first episode.

Much of the material comes from a journal I kept from 1989 onwards. For details prior to that date I have had to rely on those recollections still clear in my mind. I also circulated a questionnaire among a number of manic-depressive illness support groups around Australia, inviting members to contribute to this book by sharing some of their knowledge and experiences. Although they can in no way be representative of all the Australians suffering from this illness, their answers do serve to illustrate the human experience, and provide a far more rounded picture than if my story alone were told. Apart from my family, all names are fictitious to protect the privacy of the individuals concerned.

This book also aims to clear away some of the mysteries and fears associated not only with this illness but with psychiatry in general, and to increase understanding and tolerance among families and friends and, hopefully, the wider community.

It does not, however, claim to have all the answers, nor is it intended to be a medical reference book. Rather it provides, in easy-to-understand terms, the knowledge that I have gained, for the layperson to understand the illness, its causes and symptoms, and their treatment and management. The illness varies from person to person, and each will meet it in his or her own individual way and with varying treatment requirements. Therefore, professional treatment should always be sought, and any questions relating to the illness should be directed to the treating physician or therapist, who is the best person to give advice. This book has been written purely as an adjunct to regular treatment programs. After all, there is nothing quite like picking up a book and identifying with someone else's symptoms, be it cancer, plastic surgery or arthritis, and because manic-depressive illness is not something we tend to openly discuss, there is a need for many different avenues of support.

After eight long years, thanks to prayer, my psychiatrist and prescribed medication, my severe anguish and pain are at an end. I still experience daily fluctuations, and still have my bad days and bad weeks, but they are very mild by comparison. I do enjoy general stability now, and those around me are also able to benefit.

Natalie, who appears to have emerged from the experience the most unscathed, summed up her feelings in the following recent conversation with me:

I know that over the years we've had our ups and downs. Everybody does. But the good times definitely outnumber the bad in a huge way.

I know with your manic-depression there have been obstacles that normally wouldn't be there, and a heap of them too! I've watched you beat them for years and years with the determination and courage of a whole army. I know that sometimes I haven't made things any easier for you. It's easy to get caught up in your own thoughts and forget.

I know that I will only ever be able to see the tip of your battle, but I will always try my hardest to understand and help as best as I can.

To me, you are the most courageous, strong-willed and selfless person I know. You have been and always will be a wonderful, loving, caring mother and a great friend. Despite your manic-depression, you've supported and cared for the whole family even through the worst of it.

There have been times when the illness has made it harder for all of us, but we've stuck it out and stayed together.

I'm no expert on mental illness, but I do know that it's very real. It's also not something that you can just sleep off or take a Panadol for. It goes so deep and is so personal. It's a battle with your own mind.

I know though that, being the person you are, you will always win, and if there is anything that I can ever do, I will always be there. You might have to drum it into me at times, but I will eventually get the message. As I said before, it's easy to forget.

Tanya, who was only thirteen when the illness first struck, says she didn't understand much in the beginning or why I was taking so much medication. As she learned more about the illness, however, things did not improve for her. To the contrary, she found herself unable to accept it and blocked it out of her mind. She refused to feel anything about it, and she thinks that was possibly because she was herself depressed at the time and felt she may have a mild case of the illness. She could not deal with the possibility, no matter how remote, of being afflicted with the same illness.

Hers, too, has been a very hard road to walk.

She found it difficult to understand the concept of a mentally ill mother. She says now, 'I never thought it could have been as bad as she made it out to be. But it was.'

Gradually she says she 'came to her senses', realising there was nothing she could do but accept it and try to help me as much as she could. She says she did not feel embarrassed about the effects of the illness. But, on the other hand, she never wanted to talk about it with anyone. She was grateful that all her friends showed great understanding towards both herself and me.

Early in 1994 she said, 'It's good to see Mum on the road to recovery and, although I do not think she will ever fully recover, she is certainly getting better and there is still hope. With her strength and determination I know she can overcome the obstacles that come her way. She has always been a good friend to me and I want only the best for her, to see her as well as possible. I hope this book is very helpful for others in our position.'

George has been greatly affected because he denied it for so long. He has lost the wife he knew before the illness. He is saddened by the fact that I now find the thought of sharing his adventures uninteresting and even a source of anxiety. So George feels that he has lost his closest friend, although our relationship has improved enormously over the past twelve months into one of caring and great respect. For a long time he was mentally tired from the ordeal of trying to communicate with me over the years when I was severely depressed, having to worry about household chores and budgeting, which I used to handle capably, and at times having had the struggle of trying to keep me at home when I was high, wanting to be out having a good time.

It is easier now, of course, because my capacity to develop coping strategies, and the stabilisation of my illness to a manageable degree, have meant that he could hand back to me the general running of the household, not having to worry about the side effects of my being either severely manic or depressed, knowing that I can continue with the needs of life and fulfil my goals.

On the more positive side, the fact that George was forced to take over a number of family duties that I had always attended to has deepened and strengthened the bond between himself and Natalie and Tanya. Our marriage almost ended and this also strengthened that bond, which has been a very positive aspect that they all acknowledge.

1 Looking back

I looked down and was captivated by the beauty of the little gold heart. Uncle Joe's cold fingers were fumbling at the nape of my neck, doing up the gold chain. I shivered and snuggled closer into my daddy's arms. At the age of three, this was my first recollection of the anxiety that was part of my very essence and which would control my life. Uncle Joe's eyes were bright, his smile wide as he showed me how the locket opened, and told me softly that I could put a picture of my mummy in it. I peered at the little picture frame inside the locket. It was very special because I could hold my mummy close to me forever.

Uncle Joe's face has dimmed into oblivion now, but I still wear his little locket and treasure the memory. He wasn't my real uncle, just a kind man repaying a debt of gratitude to my father who had obtained work for him. Uncle Joe had come to live in Australia after the Second World War, and my father spent much of his time helping the migrants during those few years. In fact, my parents recently had great difficulty in remembering my Uncle Joe, let alone the locket.

Child and teenager

I was born in Sydney, but when I was three years old my father took us to live in the rural city of Albury, on the Murray River. This was the place I reluctantly called my home town from kindergarten days until I celebrated my eighteenth birthday.

As a little girl, usually dressed in blue because it highlighted my eyes and contrasted with the mop of dark curls, I fumbled and blushed my way through life, always the centre of attention, always wanting to run and hide from the admiring smiles of my mother's friends, and the prattling tongues. How I hated being the centre of attention.

Not yet five years old, I cried bitterly when I thought my mother deserted me on my first day of school. As I walked into the corridor to hang up my hat, I felt my cheeks burn. All eyes stared at me. I just knew I looked ridiculous in the green check dress and the cream straw hat that flattened my hair; and those awful gloves – they were tight, and made my hands perspire. I lowered my head and removed the hat, but once it was off there was no hiding the bright red cheeks. I wanted to just disappear, but there was no escape from the staring eyes of the horrible girls – the ones who didn't blush.

What a surprise when some of those horrible girls eventually dragged me away from the sidelines of life and forced me to join in their games. In no time at all I was giggling along with the rest of them, happy that I 'belonged'.

Eventually, the very exuberant side of my nature became apparent. My mother, on recent reflection, said that signs of a predisposition to my current illness were possibly present when I was quite young, had they only known. But who, particularly in the 1950s, would have thought of future mental illness? Who, without psychiatric knowledge, would have dreamed of looking back to their ancestry where nervous disorders, depression, even suicide, existed, to assess the mental health of their children? It was enough to cater for their usual physical and emotional needs.

So I, like many other children who eventually go on to develop this illness, was just accepted as I was, without question, but often exhausting my poor mother with my excitable nature. In her words, I had become 'a bubble ready to burst', highly strung, over-excitable and often 'high'.

I can remember constantly bursting into the kitchen like a tornado, unleashing a torrent of babble. 'Slow down, slow down,' my mother would say. 'Lower your voice an octave and slow down. I can't understand a word you're saying.' As far as I was concerned I *was* talking normally.

It has been said that personality plays a part in the occurrence of this illness, and I believe this. Personality, after all, consists of our distinctive, individual, and habitual patterns and qualities of behaviour as expressed by physical and mental activities and attitudes. It is a mixture of the temperament we are born with and the effects of subsequent experiences, and there seems little doubt that a person who is prone to shifts of mood between over-excitement and misery, combined with other predisposing factors, is more likely to develop a severe mood disorder.

Dr David Grounds and June Armstrong in their book *Ecstasy &* *Agony* state that, for reasons not yet clear, the person with an obsessional personality who is conscientious, perfectionist and predictable, is also more likely to develop major depression than people with other personality traits, though not more likely to develop the bipolar picture of mania and depression. This does not mean, of course, that *all* people of obsessional personality will develop serious depression, or that they are the only personality type that does.

There is no doubt that I was highly strung by nature, conscientious and perfectionist. I was also anxious and, although I could not express my more intangible anxieties at such a young age, I was certainly aware of many of my fears. I was afraid of the unknown, of what *might* happen if I ventured into a given situation, and I was afraid of spiders, the dark, heights and confined spaces. I always set extremely high standards for myself, particularly at school, and was always afraid that I would fall short – which probably accounted for why I was such a model student. I worried that my personal attributes were so lacking that no one could possibly like me. And, like many children, I was afraid of not living up to the expectations of my parents. So, all in all, I carried around a lot of tension.

As far back as I can remember there were two quite distinct sides to my personality: one gregarious, the other anxious, melancholy and introspective. I was rarely, if ever, on a very even keel. I often laughed too loudly, laughed till I cried, or laughed in the wrong situations, just as I often worried myself into a state of great misery. I was always drawn to melancholy music or art, to the degree that my whole outlook would be affected by haunting eyes in a picture or a soulful piece of music. It would follow me around for days. It became a part of me, and I of it, and I didn't want to let it go.

Fortunately, the gregarious side of my nature compensated for any seriousness and the load of tension that I carried, and I enjoyed lots of harmless mischief-making and the very happy times that all children enjoy.

But I often felt that somehow I was different – indeed that my whole family was strange – although I could not put my finger precisely on what that difference was. It was more than just my feelings of inadequacy; it was as though I were removed from the things of this world at times, that I did not quite belong. When I was a good deal older, I recognised part of these feelings as being my tendency to feel more deeply, think more deeply, about things that were of no interest at all to other people my own age. It was also the natural tendency I had to spend a lot of time contemplating what I thought other people were thinking, assessing their reactions, and analysing my own thoughts. Because I was so serious, adults often laughed at me and said, 'What a little old lady you are.'

Another part of this difference I felt was surely the anxiety caused by my feelings of inadequacy, and my fear of making a fool of myself. My heart thumped and my stomach churned every time I was the centre of attention. I worried about why I felt this way, why I felt inferior. Why did I place so much importance on being like others, being accepted by others? And I hated the ones who teased me about it. Someone told me I was too proud and I agonised over this one for a long time – years in fact. Did I really value myself too highly, place too much importance on myself? In the end I decided that I was aspiring to be something I was not meant to be and that I was not a very good person because of that. I stored those feelings away, but often retrieved them when I was going through a period of self-analysis. Such were the meanderings of my young mind.

I tried to bury this side of my nature, to overcome my fears, but it did not always work. Kids being kids, the stronger ones will always home in on those who are timid and give them a hard time – and I received my fair share. But I had lots of friends, and still have many happy memories of the good times, the very, very good times when our mums did tuckshop duty, the free milk, the sing-alongs on the bus trips, and the mad dash to the corner shop after school to buy a handful of broken biscuits.

Then came the extravagant yearly school operas, writing for the school magazine, and participating in eisteddfods as a pianist and cellist throughout New South Wales and Victoria.

I also remember the feelings of pride as I peered through the fence to the Catholic boys' school across the road where my father taught – and the girlish prattle and giggling as we got older, looking through the same fence at that same school, but for different reasons.

I think the best memory of home life that I carried with me into adult life was that of Mum and Dad always appearing to be so much in love. It was so important to Mum that she look her best for Dad. When he arrived home from school each day he would give her a big hug and kiss, and sweep her off her feet while she giggled. As with many families, Mum was the softie and Dad was strict. I did quite a bit of battling with him over the years, but they did everything they could to make me happy. I remember the time they sent me by train the long distance from Albury to what was then known as the Lord Mayor's Holiday Camp at Portsea, Victoria, because for some unknown reason I had been unhappy for some time and they simply did not know what to do with me. I was about eleven. That was the holiday of a lifetime, with its pillow fights and midnight snacks.

I hated my position in the family. Being the eldest of four children, I had no one to play with, as my brother was five years younger and my two sisters younger again. I often wondered if life might have been easier had I had an older brother.

My teenage years were much less anxious for me as the gregarious side of my nature took a firmer hold, but I was still highly strung and, to make matters worse, had become rebellious. Year after year Mum and Dad packed me off to Sydney or Melbourne to spend school holidays with my cousins – lazing on the beach, going out in my uncle's boat on Sydney Harbour, playing the piano, going shopping in the city.

I had learned by now to work my anxieties out of my system by various creative means, such as drawing or writing poetry or a short story. And I just loved to get into the exciting world between the covers of a good book. I read avidly, sometimes with two or three books on the go at the one time. I must have been caught a thousand times, reading under the bed covers at night by torchlight.

The biggest thing to change my world was music. At around age six I started piano lessons and soon discovered that I had a very real talent and a great love of classical music. Long before I fell in love with Elvis Presley I loved Beethoven and Mozart with a passion that I brought to life on the keyboard. My love of piano-playing grew with the years, and I discovered that if I were happy, the piano made me happier; if I were angry or sad I would vent those feelings on the piano until I had calmed down. So there was never any need for my parents to ask me to practise – I happily spent hours at the piano each night.

The piano was my comfort zone, the place where I always felt happy, in control; and it satisfied my innate need to achieve perfection. No wonder then that I achieved Honours in my exams for the next eight years, that examiners commented on my 'special gift'. I also learned the cello and played in an orchestra at various school and civic events.

Taking my nervous disposition into account, my biggest musical coup occurred when, at the age of twelve, I overcame my fears and entered a radio talent quest, despite the fact that my music teacher had forbidden me to enter. To this day I have not forgotten the buzz I got out of it, partly because I was terrified that someone would tell my teacher, and partly because I did end up being outright winner and took home a silver cup. Of course I was caught out, but I had my silver cup and that was all that mattered. The pity was that, as a result of that performance, I had been offered an opportunity to enter the world of commercial music, but I turned the offer down because I lacked confidence.

As time went by it was taken for granted that I would have a great musical career some day. I had only one more exam to do and then I would go to the Conservatorium. But, youth being what it is, I didn't have the wisdom to continue. The warmth, solace and beauty of the Masters gave way to the clatter and swing of rock 'n' roll – still I regret that decision. I rebelled against all the powers I felt were stifling me. I dropped piano lessons, thumping out rock 'n' roll instead, started going to the movies and dances in *mixed* company – strictly taboo – and defied school uniform regulations. All relatively harmless stuff, but I landed myself in a lot of hot water, both at home and at school.

So, by a very unhappy age sixteen I was ready to leave home. My parents were not very happy either. This new era of rock 'n' roll was difficult for strict Catholic parents to cope with – much the way I found discos worrying when my daughters first started going out. But we battled on, and although things settled down somewhat, I eventually left home at age eighteen and moved to Melbourne. My mother came with me and helped me find accommodation and a job, her dear face etched with worry lines, the tone of her voice echoing her fears. But I knew a sense of relief. I needed to be alone, to experience life and learn from my own experiences, to put what I saw as a troubled life behind me. Now I could be happy, mistress of my own destiny, living in a boarding house and settled into a job in a law firm.

At last there was relative calm in my life. But that was the calm before the storm, the storm that overshadowed my life for several years, and made my rebellious years pale into insignificance.

Life away from home

I was suddenly jerked into groggy consciousness, my mind drifting back towards oblivion again, my eyes too heavy to open. My body seemed a long way away, as though it didn't belong to me.

A voice was yelling, and my eyes stirred unwillingly. Both my arms were suddenly yanked sharply, and a feeble anger stirred deep within me. But the anger didn't last – the voice faded away, and I sank back into the welcome darkness.

Again I heard the voice, louder this time, and my arms were being yanked again, more sharply. But still I did not want to wake up, and I wished the voice away.

'Come on, walk,' it yelled in my ear. 'Stop dragging those feet.'

My chin was resting on my chest. I formed a tiny slit with one eye and peered down at the floor. Even though I could not see it clearly, it did not seem familiar. I saw feet on either side of me. Two people, holding me up between them, with my arms around their necks. There were two voices now, and I could hear them quite clearly. The anger stirred again.

'I'm too tired,' I mumbled. 'Just leave me alone. I want to go to sleep.'

'If you go to sleep you'll probably never wake up again,' one of the voices said. 'You're lucky to be here, you know. Now put those feet on the ground, one in front of the other, and walk.' The voice was stern, with a tone of urgency.

They nudged my legs. 'Come on,' the voice persisted. 'Walk.'

They pulled my arms again and my eyes opened. I saw heavy shoes, and uniforms. Policewomen. I shuffled, struggling to lift my wobbly legs, the policewomen carrying most of my weight. My mind was constantly drifting off.

They ignored my pleas to be left alone, kept nudging my legs and pulling on my arms as we walked, every step an effort. After a while we sat down and they helped me swallow some coffee. This procedure went on and on. Walking, more walking, then a drink.

Hazy memories of bottles of pills finally came to mind, and I suddenly realised they had saved my life.

This episode took place in the early 1960s, in my late teenage years. To this day I do not know if that overdose was deliberate or accidental, and whether or not I was affected by the same highs and lows that I have recently experienced as a result of my manic-depressive disorder, one that does appear during teenage years, and which can definitely result in suicide attempts. Today I can only speculate about these things but, taking my whole life and my personality into consideration, it seems possible that I was affected by illness at that time. Without doubt my moods were excessively high and low, and I did things then that I would never have considered doing during my 'rebellious days'.

During that turbulent period I used alcohol excessively when my spirits were unduly high, then barbiturates from an endless number of doctors to procure the sleep and peace of mind that often eluded me for long periods. Then I turned to 'uppers' to keep me going through times of excessive sleep and lethargy. I remember having a lot of trouble obtaining those magic pills that I came to rely upon so heavily. The moment a doctor started asking too many questions, trying to pinpoint my problem, I was off like a shot to another, worrying (without knowing exactly why) that they would find something wrong with me that I would not want to know about.

In those days, of course, the question of illness, particularly mental illness, would never have entered my mind. I often wondered why I behaved the way I did, but simply put it down to an unwanted flaw in my character – I had been tarred with the devil's brush, so to speak, and thought it was all part of my feelings of being 'different'. I was actually a very unhappy young woman. But mental illness was not something one even thought about, let alone talked about, belonging as it did to a world of *other* people, not *my* world.

That period eventually passed, of course, and I stepped back into a conventional lifestyle, forming a new life for myself, with nobody knowing anything about those times. The feelings of guilt and shame, however, remained with me, and it is only recently that I have been able to come to terms with my past.

I assume that my abuse of alcohol and medication have blotted out much of that short period of my life forever, but I still have some very vivid memories that will never leave me. Life was one big roller coaster, outrageously soaring on the highs, then hitting low spots where I turned away from friends because of general feelings of fear and unreality. Other images also come to mind of being huddled up, cradling my head, depressed.

There seems little doubt that all the features of manic-depressive illness were present. When my mood was high I was over-exuberant, did not sleep normally, spent enormous amounts of money and had a libido that refused to subside. My parents paid many of my debts. For quite some time I moved from job to job, completely unsettled – at times unhappy, at times out raging, but never keeping friends or jobs for long.

My teenage years behind me, I settled into a flat in inner suburban Melbourne with a very conventional and traditionally minded friend from a small country town. I still felt emotionally unbalanced, prone to anxiety, some depressive moods and, at times, somewhat outrageous behaviour, albeit greatly toned down from what it had been. I was by now very good at hiding my unbalanced nature, so in me my friend saw a conscientious, dedicated, caring person who had an enormous zest for life. The qualities we each brought into the friendship seemed to complement the other's very nicely.

In my early twenties I met George, son of a former Polish solicitor. Four years my senior, he was mature, stable, and intelligent, working in the area of industrial chemistry. He was very well-read with a quick, keen mind, and I found his companionship stimulating, a welcome change from the type of men with whom I had previously associated. We spent many long hours talking each week and soon became firm friends. Without realising it initially, I began to lean on him for emotional stability and security, and then fell madly in love with him.

By the time we were married just before my twenty-third birthday, most of my inner turmoil had subsided. My behaviour still tended to be unacceptable from time to time but was now tempered by a great desire to settle down, raise a family, and lead a quieter life, which was very quickly achieved. Within five years we were blessed with two beautiful daughters, Natalie and Tanya.

Until early 1986 we shared a very spacious double-storey bluestone home with George's widowed mother Aleksandra in Melbourne's historic suburb of Williamstown. Well-educated, intelligent and sensitive, Aleksandra was a fount of strength and wisdom to all who knew her. With her help Natalie and Tanya learned to speak fluent Polish. Due to a large family business loss, I had to continue working whilst Aleksandra looked after the girls each day until I returned home from work.

Aleksandra, having spent her life as a professional artist, opened a studio in our home and taught many people including myself, Natalie and Tanya, how to see life through the eyes of an artist, and we shared with her the joy of creating life on canvas while she watched us reap the rewards that can be gained only through dedication and self-discipline.

Art became an all-consuming passion for me. I organised community art shows, sold my paintings and sketches, and eventually was being commissioned to do work for a number of people. This was wonderful at a time when I could see my talents finally beginning to emerge, and it was a way of developing my skills even further. However, the desire to create, to paint for others, and to constantly aim for perfection, was taking me over. No longer content with two to three hours' painting and sketching each night, I began spending six to eight hours at the easel each night, often until two in the morning. It had become all or nothing, and so I eventually had to lay down my pens and brushes to devote myself entirely to my family and my job.

My history of ill health included a number of surgical procedures, and many stress-induced disorders, some of which lasted for many years. From my early twenties onwards I continually read books that dealt with stress, self-esteem and confidence. I tried yoga, acupuncture and relaxation tapes but, whilst I developed a greater awareness of my inner problems, harmony and balance continued to elude me. What I did gain over a period of time was enormous patience and tolerance in almost any situation, and the determination to pursue and achieve goals that were important to me.

Having suffered from a manic-depressive disorder now for about eight years, it is no wonder that I have turned the clock back to piece together the jigsaw of my life. Were those earlier years the beginning of the illness? Have there been other milder episodes since, when my behaviour was certainly somewhat unbalanced? I wonder. It would certainly explain a lot of things, such as my need to seek medical help for my problems.

I doubt I shall ever know for sure, and it does not matter too much any more. But at times it mattered greatly, because the troubled mind hates such questions left unanswered, like an unsolved crime. It prefers to have them neatly packaged, labelled 'complete', then tidily stored away in the archives. But my search is now over, and the memories, less painful, have again been stored away.

Why should the softest whisper
Be as thunder to my ear,
Or the tree's inviting shadow
Send me scurrying in fear.

Catherine Rzecki

2 The onset of my illness

Spring had suddenly emerged, leaving the leaden skies and bitter winds of winter far behind.

There was another wind brewing silently now. Not the wind that smacks the cheeks and picks up the leaves, but a whirlwind silently gathering force and stirring at the innermost recesses of my mind. I was blissfully unaware of this storm brewing within, unaware that it would soon bring madness and mayhem into my life and the lives of those around me.

For each of us, it is only the face of the storm that varies, be it death, illness, financial problems or rifts in family relationships. For our family at this time, it was my unexpected and bewildering mental illness, which first manifested itself as anxiety.

I will never forget the soft, balmy day in 1987 when I experienced my first anxiety attack. There was a sweetness in the air that only spring can bring. I was in good spirits. And why shouldn't I be? I'd had a cancerous melanoma removed earlier that year and I knew I was lucky to be alive. I had been told that had I ignored the little pink mole on my leg for another six months, I might not have lived to enjoy another springtime. A chilling thought at the time, but one that now left me at peace with my God and myself.

As I left the office that day and started my daily walk to the bank, the vibrant air announced that the sluggishness of winter had finally been shed. People seemed to be walking taller with a new vitality, and there were splashes of colour on trees and in garden beds. Definitely not a day for working, I thought, as I took a deep breath and forged ahead. I could not allow myself the luxury of dwelling too long on the pleasantness of the day because I was running late and had to catch the bank before it closed.

Being in a hurry, however, didn't stop me calling out to the greengrocer as I rushed past his shop. After working in the area almost two years I knew a lot of the locals and felt very comfortable with them. In fact, I loved Carlisle Street with its incongruous mix of people. The population was mostly transient, from countries all over the world, laced with the flavour that only nearby St Kilda could bring. In stark contrast a more sober note was added by the liberal sprinkling of men from the local Jewish community, outstanding in their black garb, long beards and black hats.

I bolted into the bank moments before the doors were closed, thankful for the few minutes of peace and quiet while my money was being counted. I took a deep breath, and was soon on my way back to the office.

Suddenly I became aware of a new stillness in the air, and the noise of the tram rolling by was irritatingly loud. It left me with an unpleasant feeling of unreality, a momentary feeling that something was amiss, followed by a quick sensation of fear that disappeared just as swiftly as it had come.

Then, just as suddenly I felt lightheaded and very sluggish and my heart skipped a beat. I ran my hand across my moist forehead, noticing at the same time that my throat and lips were very dry. I was puzzled, wondering why I should suddenly feel so tired and ill. Perhaps I was coming down with a cold?

That feeling of unreality, I now know, is caused by nervous tension and is quite common. At the time, however, I became more tense, more anxious, steeling myself against these unpleasant sensations. Within minutes I was dizzy and nauseated, my heart thumped loudly and painfully in my throat, and my vision was blurred. The pavement seemed suddenly to dip and sway away from me. I felt faint, wanting to vomit, and my legs wobbled.

Somehow I stumbled across the pavement and steadied myself against a shop-front, frightened, bewildered, and embarrassed. What if someone I knew had seen me? I composed myself as best I could, then continued slowly, head down, hugging the walls and fences along the way. It didn't happen again, but I couldn't dismiss the feeling of unease all the way back to the office.

Back at work I had a glass of water and decided to put the episode out of my mind. Obviously I had been rushing around too much and neglecting meals – I wouldn't let it happen again. But it did, the next day, with such intensity that I was forced to seek help from a shopkeeper. The pavement seemed to be falling away in front of my eyes, and on top of all the other symptoms I was now gasping for air and my lips and fingers were numb. Terrified, I somehow made my way into a shop where the concerned shopkeeper gave me a seat and a glass of water and chatted to me until I was more composed. I tried to pass it off to her as something trivial, but I was feeling deeply uneasy.

Had I gone to a doctor that day, I would have been told that the difficulty with breathing was caused by hyperventilating (overbreathing in fright) which resulted in the numbness in my lips and fingers. I would also have been told that all the other symptoms were manifestations of anxiety, and could be treated. But I did not see a doctor.

I thought about the possible causes of the attacks and came up with two possibilities, both remote. One was a brain tumour, the other stress. The idea of a tumour played on my mind for some time, but I did not want to rush off to a doctor until I had given myself a reasonable chance to 'will' the problem away. And if indeed it *was* a tumour I was not at all certain that I would want to hear that diagnosis anyway.

So I allowed the 'attacks' to persist with relentless ferocity, each more intense than the last, and always on the way to or from the bank, which seemed odd. Because it was happening mid-afternoon, I thought it might have something to do with my not eating enough during the day, so I started eating larger, more nutritious lunches, and stopped rushing around so much, but those measures proved unhelpful.

Eventually I began to feel completely unnerved. My body seemed somehow detached and I watched, terrified, as my other self floundered, my head flooding with moments of dimming consciousness.

I soon decided to go via the back streets to the bank, to avoid embarrassment. I continued this way for some time, with people often stopping to offer help. I recall one day in particular, when I thought I had reached the end of my tether. I was leaning against a wall, squatting with my head down, trying to summon enough strength to carry on, when I felt a hand on my shoulder. I looked up into the dirty face of an old man who probably had not washed or shaved in weeks.

'You OK love?' His raspy voice sounded distant somehow.

I decided he was harmless enough – the drink had obviously seen to that – but his odour was as offensive as the dirty old khaki coat with its bulging pockets. But at least he had stopped, I thought. At least he had brought me back to reality for a moment.

I mustered a weak smile and stood up slowly, my legs still wobbly.

'Yes thanks, I'm OK.'

'Ya need help?' He extended a dirty hand.

'No. I'll be all right now. Thanks for stopping.'

It was not only his smell that brought me back to reality. It was my amazement that such a person would bother to stop. But his concern was real, even if it was smothered in alcohol.

Looking back now, I wonder why on earth I did not see a doctor at that stage. But I made a deliberate decision not to. I was going to beat this 'thing', burying my fears behind a wall of fierce determination, and praying with more fervour than ever for the help I needed.

The attacks continued, no longer confined to my trips to the bank. Waiting in a queue at the bank or the checkout queue at the supermarket soon became times to dread. Often in the bank queue I thought I was going to pass out, and on a number of occasions I had to ask for help. I asked the person ahead of me to hold my bankbooks until she reached the head of the queue, explaining that I wasn't well, and I sat down to wait my turn. It was a little easier being seated. I really did not care too much that people witnessed this – it was much better than collapsing in an unsightly heap on the floor. Outside the bank I could eventually relax a bit. Once I was able to take a few deep breaths I could continue on my unsteady way.

Everywhere I went, I was anticipating a panic attack, and before I went out anywhere I would always have carefully planned my 'escape route', plus what I would do if *this* happened, or if *that* happened.

I felt ashamed, guilty, and frightened of being branded an 'oddity' by anyone who witnessed my failings. I wanted to tell someone but how could I explain what I did not understand myself? No one could possibly understand such irrational behaviour. I was no longer the person I used to be, and I began to wonder whether I ever would be again.

The walks to and from the bank continued to be the most distressing, and eventually I had to drive the short distance to Carlisle Street. That didn't help either. My first major attack in the car was terrifying – I seemed to have lost all control of my actions and rationality, and a terrible accident seemed inevitable.

It was towards the end of that year of 1987 when the attacks took a turn for the worse. I was driving home from work over the Westgate Bridge when the road ahead suddenly seemed to fade away. My legs shook uncontrollably and I found it difficult to keep my foot on the pedal. I felt violently ill, my head was swimming, and I could not focus on anything around me. Gasping for breath, my hands and fingers numb and shaking, I crawled into the left lane, sure that I would black out at any moment. The traffic noises were thunderous, and cars seemed to be rocketing by, leaving me standing still in my own world of fear. Feeling completely disoriented, I moved into the emergency lane, slowing down to a crawl, praying that I would not black out.

Suddenly a searing pain flashed through my body, leaving all the nerve endings throbbing with the prickly pain that runs up the back of the neck after a terrible fright, except that this was much more intense. It was quickly followed by another surge, leaving me with the feeling that I had experienced an electric shock. Somehow I hobbled home, stopping every so often, arriving weak and exhausted, but thankful to be alive. There was no doubt in my mind that I was just as dangerous on the road as a person who is very drunk.

That night, thoughts of the incident triggered memories from my past – memories that should have sent me scurrying to a doctor. About six years earlier I'd been involved in a nasty highway accident. The car flipped over and over, hitting a pole and ending up on the median strip facing in the opposite direction. Luckily we were not hurt, but were shocked, and out of that accident I lost my confidence and developed a traffic phobia that necessitated psychotherapy before I could drive confidently again. My symptoms now were very similar to those I experienced then – only much much worse.

Once again I tested my previously learned behaviour therapy techniques, but found they did not work. By now I felt very threatened and, for the first time, actually *recognised* panic in my reactions. I constantly visualised myself and my children being carried away from the scene of an accident, and saw myself completely 'flipped out', having no control at all over my mind or body.

The thought of a respite from driving during the forthcoming Christmas vacation was the only thing that kept me going at that time. Surely the month's break would cure me. But the constant battle was quickly exhausting me, and one day at work a colleague found me slumped in a chair, my head in my hands. I sobbed uncontrollably as she tried to comfort me, assuring me that it was bound to be stress, and easily remedied. My husband, George, was called to take me to a doctor.

My doctor was overseas at the time, so I saw an associate, a quietly spoken, fatherly type who told me gently that I was suffering from anxiety. His explanation suggested a nervous condition.

I stared in disbelief. 'You mean it's just a nervous condition?' I asked, searching his face for confirmation.

His reply in the affirmative was good news, and he sounded so sure that I simply had to believe him. If it was a nervous condition, then it was definitely something I could sink my teeth into and overcome. Hadn't I always? He prescribed the tranquilliser oxazepam (Serepax), which I had never had before, and advised me to rest. Unfortunately, he neglected to explain the nature of anxiety and panic attacks, so I left his surgery thinking I was dealing with a *simple* nervous condition.

It would have helped had I been told that my nervous responses were the usual responses to stress but greatly exaggerated; that they were heightened each time I experienced fear, anxiety or dread of the symptoms to the point where I had an 'attack of panic', the most alarming and sensitising of all the symptoms. I should also have been told that, because of my continual agitation, my nerves were in a constant state of alarm, that I was, in fact, adding stress to the original stress each time I registered fear of the symptoms, thus placing myself on a merry-go-round of tension–fear–tension–fear.

Had the doctor explained these things to me, perhaps in time I could have learned to face the fear and overcome it with relaxation, instead of trying to fight it. I eventually learned, with experience, that 'fighting' it only adds to the problem because of the added tension involved.

I took the Serepax faithfully and waited for the attacks to stop, fully expecting medication, combined with my indomitable spirit, to do the job. Certainly the attacks eased, but they did not disappear. Without even realising it, I was watching for any sign of the symptoms recurring, and in doing so I became more tense; and so the attacks persisted, with less severity, but still surviving in their bed of tension.

Another source of tension for me was that I had difficulty explaining my feelings to my family, and the close friends I wished to confide in. Only those who have experienced a panic attack can really understand the fear and pain, and any attempt at explanation sounded absurd.

I decided to adopt a more positive attitude, and borrowed some books on stress and relaxation from the local library – one book in particular by Dr Ainslie Meares, which had helped me through some difficult periods in the past. With this new attitude, I felt sure I would soon be living life to the full once again. I soon discovered, however, that it was not to be so easy.

The symptoms reappeared whilst I was sitting in the church one Sunday, and I felt hundreds of staring eyes on my back as I gasped painfully and embarrassingly for air. I had to leave the church, and from that day on I always sat at the end of the back pew, close to the door, ready for a quick exit when necessary. The same thing happened in theatres and restaurants, school concerts and meetings – anywhere in fact where I felt 'trapped' in confined spaces, with too many people, or where I was not close to the exit.

But driving caused the most enormous physical and emotional distress, and each time I felt I was becoming too hazardous on the road I increased the dosage of Serepax. The effects of each increased dosage would last only a short while, so it was not long before I seemed to be swallowing them like lollies, not realising how difficult it would be to give them up later on. That was another point the doctor had not made – how easy it is to become dependent, and how painful are the withdrawal symptoms. I was to discover that for myself many months later.

Few people realised the extent of my problem because I concealed it well. It is amazing how cunning we become when we have something to conceal – something that causes us shame or embarrassment – and my predicament caused me a good deal of both. Once an energetic person shouldering a lot of responsibilities, I was now reduced to a quivering lump, afraid of my own shadow but not knowing why. One by one, each strategy that I adopted crumbled around me, destroying all my self-confidence. I avoided all driving and social engagements that were not absolutely essential, developing an endless list of excuses to avoid exposure.

I remember when I was a youngster, all nervous disorders were referred to as 'nerves'. I remember hearing the 'oldies' saying such things as 'But he suffers from nerves, you know' with a knowing and sympathetic nod. Well, 'nerves' ran through both sides of our family, and I don't expect to be any different. In fact we've always been able to joke about it, aunts, uncles, cousins, the lot. The big difference for me was that, for the first time, I had not been able to gain any control over my problem, and I was completely bewildered.

I did recognise at that point, however, that I was suffering from nervous fatigue, a condition involving physical, emotional and mental fatigue. I did not understand, of course, how or why it had developed, although I soon learned that it creeps up in such an insidious manner that the nervously ill person doesn't recognise what is happening.

A possible example is a person who begins feeling very tired, then later on goes on to experience some of the slightly exaggerated symptoms mentioned earlier; she then becomes afraid of the condition she's in, thinking that these distressing symptoms have a physiological cause. When it persists and worsens, she may begin to think she is going crazy, so adding stress to stress. She remains totally unaware that these symptoms are caused by fatigue, and that, when fatigued, nerves become so aroused that they register emotions more acutely, building up to the point where an ordinary flash of fear is felt as a painful spasm of panic – the type of 'electric shock' that I had been experiencing.

Lack of understanding leads to more distress, more fear than ever, so adding more stress-fear to the original stress-fear. The mind tends to dwell on the illness all the time, in a fruitless attempt to discover the cause and eradicate the problem, and so concentration is impaired.

At this point, all other emotions can register more intensely too – an ordinary joke might cause hysterical laughter, an unhappy event might seem tragic, and everyday noises, such as traffic, can seem so thunderous and distorted that the person may feel disoriented and have to escape from the area of the noise.

I was now in such a position, and I decided to visit the doctor again. He was alarmed at the amount of Serepax I was taking and asked me to slowly reduce the quantity. As it happened, he also practised hypnotherapy, and suggested a few sessions, although he could not guarantee they would work. I agreed. I would have agreed to anything at that stage.

Hypnotherapy sessions started straight away, and I was also given a relaxation tape to use before sleeping. I was relieved that I was now able to take further positive steps to help myself, feeling sure that this time my problem could be conquered. Every night I went to bed a little earlier, using the tape to try to relax. On weekends I used it morning and night. Having used similar tapes successfully in the past, I should have been able to relax both physically and mentally, but I simply could not 'let go'.

The hypnotherapy sessions were not what I was expecting, and I was disappointed right from the start that I did not respond well. I was asked to lie down on a couch where I made myself as comfortable as I could, considering that my nerves were stretched taut. The doctor then 'talked me down' in stages, from a level of high nervous arousal to one where I should have been almost asleep. In soothing tones, his voice led me from my agitated state of consciousness, down, down, down, to a place where my body and mind should have been flooded with peace and warmth – a place where I could rest undisturbed. But I could not reach it because of palpitations and overbreathing, and on the few occasions when I had just stepped into this beautiful place, the panic response was triggered and I started hyperventilating badly. Each session left me feeling more and more concerned for my future well-being. I felt this 'thing', whatever it was, was with me to stay.

Christmas holidays were a welcome relief that year. I cancelled all appointments except my hypnotherapy sessions and going to church, and did only the barest minimum of driving. I wanted to give both my body and my mind a complete rest, hoping to be completely well again when I returned to work in 1988.

Each time I went to a hypnotherapy session it was only a twenty-minute drive from home, but every trip was a real test of endurance and, dare I say it, courage. I could not drive over thirty kilometres an hour. Even doing forty I felt like a rocket hurtling out of control. Everything – the kerb, the lines on the road, the passing traffic – seemed to be speeding around me at such a threatening pace that my head was reeling. If I kept the window closed, I felt claustrophobic; if I opened it the traffic noise was so exaggerated to my sensitive hearing that I became completely disoriented. It was impossible to feel safe and in control behind the wheel. In fact, I was not in control, not safe.

Hypnotherapy sessions continued through the Christmas holidays and beyond, into 1988. But there was no relief. The panic states had become a way of life. I was overwhelmed by a continual state of intense fear, of anything, everything, and nothing in particular. Just this constant terrifying fear, eating away at me. I hyperventilated day and night until I forgot what it was like to breathe normally, always terrified that I might pass out. I resisted the Serepax as much as possible, but eventually found myself increasing the dosage just so that I could carry on with life. I was tired and miserable, afraid to leave the safety and comfort of my home.

I very clearly remember my first day back at work. I was in a panic of sorts even before I left the house. As I closed the back door behind me, my heart skipped a beat and I could taste the fear. Painful memories of past attacks flashed before my eyes, so I switched to relaxation mode, mentally and physically, filling my mind with the most relaxing and pleasing pictures I could conjure up. I focused all my attention on these pictures as I walked to the car.

Behind the wheel, before I had even taken the car out of the garage, the pictures kept slipping away as the fear took over. I became lightheaded, and every nerve ending was standing up and tingling, just like the hairs on the back of my neck after a fright. I tried to think ahead, to plan my day at the office, to relax and ignore the pain.

I turned into the main road ahead, and a wave of fear surged through me like a 240-volt current. The pain left me weak and trembling, and all my nerve endings pulsated with a prickling pain. I stayed in the left-hand lane, trying to compose myself. 'Calm down, just relax,' I said. 'It hasn't killed you yet.'

I checked the rear-vision mirror. There was a car close behind me, and the driver was narrowing the gap between our vehicles. I wanted him to pass because I needed to drive slowly without the pressure of knowing I was slowing him down. I was still very lightheaded and frightened, and everything around me seemed to be flashing by at great speed, as on a race-track. Another surge of fear, then another, and the sharp pain drained me of energy. I couldn't think clearly any more. I began to panic, breathing too quickly, my heart pounding.

How on earth would I get to work? I wanted to pull over, but as usual I struggled on, shaking violently but determined not to give in. I crawled onto the Westgate Bridge, but when I reached the top I was overcome by a fear of the great height, the seemingly endless stretch of road, and the speed of the traffic. I was shaking uncontrollably, terrified that I would black out behind the wheel. I reached for the Serepax, always on the car seat. At least it might calm me down a bit by the time I arrived at work.

I made it to work, as I always did, wondering what my future held. Would hypnotherapy eventually work for me? I doubted it very much. If not, what alternatives were there? Where does one go when the doctors don't have the answers?

Was it patience or a sense of helplessness that kept me going to hypnotherapy sessions for the next couple of months? Then one night as I lay on the doctor's couch, trying desperately not to hyperventilate, he stopped the hypnotherapy session and said, 'I really don't think this is working, do you?'

I felt like screaming, 'I could have told you that months ago!' but sitting up on the couch I simply asked in desperation, 'Where do we go from here, Doctor?' For the first time in my life I was unable to help myself, even with assistance, so I was relying on him to have all the answers.

'Well, my dear, I think you're suffering from depression.' His fatherly face broke into an apologetic half-smile. 'I'd like to try you on some anti-depressant medication.'

'What?' I almost laughed in his face. It seemed like some sort of cruel joke. 'No, you're wrong,' I said firmly. 'I'm not depressed.' How could he possibly suggest such a thing? Sure, life didn't appear too bright at the moment, but that was to be expected after all I'd been through.

'Well, I'd like you to try some antidepressants anyway – I think they could help you. Besides,' he added, 'they'll help you sleep.'

That would be a pleasant change, but what medication could possibly be prescribed for feeling miserable? A tranquilliser to promote sleep? I was desperate enough to try anything. I sank back into the couch and closed my eyes while he wrote out a prescription. What on earth would I do if the antidepressants didn't help me?

He explained that while there could be some side effects such as dry mouth and dizziness, they should not interfere with my life. But I was in no way prepared for the side effects as I took my first dose of imipramine (Tofranil) that night before going to bed. They were so severe that I thought surely he must have prescribed the wrong medication. I lay down, drowsy and apprehensive. Then my vision blurred, and when I could no longer clearly see the other side of the room I started to panic. I sat up on the bed, the room spinning violently. I feared that if I put my head on the pillow I might never wake again. Cautiously I slid off the bed. I had to move, to do something positive.

I squatted on the floor, weeping tears of anger and distress. What was this doctor doing to me? How could he do this after all I had been through? I picked up the packet of Tofranil but couldn't even read the print because of my distorted vision. Still crying bitterly, I managed to crawl to the toilet, where I flushed all the capsules away.

I called out to George, frightened and in need of moral support. Seeing me in this condition, he was first alarmed, then furious. How could my problem have got so out of hand that a doctor was now prescribing such drugs? We agreed that it was totally unwarranted.

I fought against the medication as long as I could that night, too frightened to turn out the light. George finally became a bit exasperated.

'Don't worry – they're not going to kill you,' he said. 'Turn the light out and get some sleep.' I eventually succumbed to the whirling darkness and had my first good night's sleep in a long, long time.

The next morning I woke up, groggy but thankful to be alive. I was in such a state of anger and despair I could not go to work. As soon as I was alert enough, I rang the doctor and berated him.

'I'm so sorry,' he said, obviously stunned by my violent outburst. 'I've never known Tofranil to have such an effect. You'd better not take any more.'

'Don't worry,' I said, angry and shaking. 'I flushed them all down the toilet last night.'

I had wasted enough time with him. I decided there and then that I would go back to my regular doctor. But looking back, I would have to say that I was simply unlucky enough to have had a particularly bad reaction to Tofranil. What I did not know at that time was that I actually *was* slipping into depression, and was really in need of psychiatric help.

It was now well into 1988, and my regular doctor kept me on a reduced dose of Serepax plus nitrazepam (Mogadon) for sleeping. He was very understanding, but very firm about continually reducing the Serepax. I could not do it. Each time I tried reducing the dosage, the anxiety and panic attacks increased alarmingly. I did not know then that withdrawal symptoms often present themselves in the same physical form as anxiety symptoms, making it difficult at times to differentiate between the two.

My doctor and I dug deep into my personal life to find anything that could have triggered my anxiety, but we always came up empty-handed. He felt it was a general anxiety state, not specifically related to traffic. I agreed, but other than that we were at a loss. I came to the conclusion that there must be something locked away in my mind that I could not recognise. My constant terror was eating into my physical and mental well-being more and more, and my body needed a rest, to be bathed in peace and quiet for a time.

I said to my doctor one day, 'This problem is obviously anxiety, but it's been going on far too long and we can't find a reason, so I'd like to see a specialist and try to get to the bottom of it.'

'You want to see a psychiatrist, then?' he asked.

'Yes,' I replied firmly. 'There seems no point in wasting any more time. If there's something locked away in my mind that started this anxiety, then I should be seeing someone qualified to help me find out what it is.'

He agreed, and I asked for a referral to Dr W., the psychiatrist who had helped me after the car accident. I liked and trusted him because he had been opposed to using drugs and had cured my problem using only psychotherapy. I felt confident that if anyone could help me get to the bottom of this problem and wean me off the Serepax, he could.

And so I left the surgery, clinging to my referral and to a new glimmer of hope.

Our Father knows what's best for us,
So why should we complain –
We always want the sunshine,
But He knows there must be rain

Helen Steiner Rice

3 A diagnosis of depression

My psychiatrist

My psychiatrist! No matter how many other patients he has, Dr W. will always be my psychiatrist. How can it be otherwise when he's been privy to my innermost thoughts, my deepest secrets, which no other being will ever know? Like all patients, I soon developed a strong attachment to my doctor, because he held my very life in the palm of his hand. Over the years he continuously monitored my physical well-being and guided me through years of darkness and mental aberration. He was the only one who understood my plight, to whom I could turn without fear of rejection or disapproval.

While he offered guidance, support and counselling, he was never judgmental as I poured out my fears, shame and guilt. When I was bogged down in past or present darkness, he gently pointed the way to the future. He was always available to me, day or night, never complaining. To him, it was simply a matter of doing his job, but he always did that in such a professional and compassionate manner that he earned my trust and respect immediately. So, he will always be *my* psychiatrist, no matter how many other patients say the same thing.

On that unforgettable first visit in June 1988, my emotions were in turmoil, a mixture of relief, apprehension and impatience. By that time I was certainly feeling depressed, although I did not recognise the depression for what it would ultimately turn out to be.

Thankfully there were only a couple of people in the waiting room, or I could not have sat through the waiting period without hyperventilating. As it was, my toes wiggled up and down frantically to relieve the tension, and my breathing became fast and shallow as my panic gradually mounted. The other patients looked very ordinary, like myself, and I wondered what had brought them to a psychiatrist. Were they really ill, or just suffering some simple complaint like my own? There was almost a touch of the ridiculous in seeing a psychiatrist about a nervous disorder – after all, I was not mentally ill, was I? But I reminded myself that no one else had been able to help me, and that was why I was here.

Time dragged while I leafed through a couple of magazines, looking vacantly at the pictures but not reading a word. As my tension grew, so did the feeling of being trapped, and I began hyperventilating, knowing that soon I would have to rush outside into the fresh air.

'Catherine Rzecki.' My name came floating smoothly across the room, putting an instant brake on the tension.

Dr W. stood in the doorway, and I crossed the room towards his outstretched hand. His grip was firm and reassuring, putting me instantly at ease. I imagine he must learn a lot from his patients through that initial handshake. He ushered me into his room, and I was envious of his calm, self-assured bearing. He didn't seem to have changed at all since I last saw him except for a few grey hairs noticeable against his olive skin.

We sat down, and he smiled, his dark eyes seeming to penetrate the very depths of my being. He talked quietly, reminding me of the previous success we had had with my traffic phobia.

'Have you had any further problems with your driving?' he asked.

'No, none at all,' I said, assuring him that his work with me had been successful. 'Well, until recently that is,' I added.

'Oh? Would you like to tell me about it?' He smiled.

With relief I poured it all out. He then quizzed me about other things that seemed irrelevant to me but were obviously important to him, such as my inability to concentrate, loss of confidence, loss of interest in life generally, and insomnia. The questions kept coming. I looked at him, suddenly anxious. We seemed to be going off at a tangent here, and I had no idea where we were headed.

He then asked about my relationship with George and our two daughters, followed by a myriad of questions about my life from childhood to the present. This seemed more appropriate – maybe in the maze of my lifetime we could find some reason for my anxiety. I had certainly had my share of emotional storms over the years, and there could be something locked away as a result.

He pressed on, bringing my medical history up to date, uncovering previous anxieties and a couple of bouts of mild depression. Then he asked for the medical history of all my relatives. 'All of them, aunts, uncles, grandparents – the lot,' he said.

This was difficult, particularly with mental and emotional disorders, because I was vague about the precise nature of such disturbances in the more extended family. I knew that there were nervous disorders on both sides of the family, that there was one instance of depression but I had no idea of how severe, and that there were two breakdowns, one of those persons still being ill after ten years.

Head down, he took copious notes until finally he seemed satisfied that he had everything he needed. He sat back in his chair for a moment before speaking, and again my toes started working furiously. What would he say? Where would we go from here? I prayed to God not to desert me.

Finally came the verdict, delivered like a kindly judge handing down a difficult sentence. 'Well, my dear, you are suffering from depression, what we call endogenous depression.' His voice was clear and firm – there was obviously no doubt in his mind.

I skipped over the word endogenous for the moment. 'But I don't see *why* I should be depressed,' I interrupted. 'Except that the anxiety has understandably made me a bit miserable.'

'Please – let me explain what endogenous depression is,' he said. 'Endogenous means "from within" – that is, your depression is not a reaction to external events, but rather it comes from within you yourself. There are genetic and biochemical factors involved.' He went on to explain how chemical imbalances occurred within the brain, while I listened, dumbfounded. He was telling me that I was ill – and mentally ill at that! I had not come to hear this. I was just an ordinary person, and ordinary people do not become mentally ill, out of the blue. It simply was not possible. I could not accept it.

'But I still don't understand,' I said, trying to look as calm as possible. 'I'm quite obviously suffering from anxiety. Look at the traffic phobia and the constant hyperventilating!' I was fighting for my life here, and I would have to try to prove him wrong.

'Yes, this type of depression is often accompanied by anxiety, and often it's the anxiety we see first.'

'But how do you know it's this type of depression?' I kept pushing, still not satisfied.

He explained that, as with physical illness, certain symptoms must be present to enable such a diagnosis to be made. If there is no obvious external cause for the depth of depression and the symptoms have been present for a long time, as they had with me, then a diagnosis of endogenous depression must be made, particularly when there is any family history of depression. The symptoms included the things we had been talking about – loss of interest in what used to give pleasure, insomnia with early morning wakening and agitation, poor concentration, loss of libido and a general feeling of depressed mood.

'And there is no possibility at all that some problem in my personal life is responsible?' I asked, feeling quite dazed.

His 'no' was sympathetic but firm.

What could I say? I really trusted this man, and even though the whole thing sounded quite absurd, I somehow knew I had to accept what he had told me. But how difficult it was to digest! Within the space of a moment my status in life had changed from 'average person' to that of someone who bore the stigma of mental illness. And all I had wanted was for this man to find some emotional problem that I could overcome quickly.

'How long is it likely to last?' At least there might be some hope here.

'Well, I will start you on some antidepressant medication. It takes a few weeks to start working, but then you should notice a marked improvement.' His tone sounded positive, until he added, 'But there is sometimes a bit of difficulty finding just the right medication for each individual. What works well for one person might not for someone else – so we may have to try a couple before we find the one that works best for you.'

This did not sound quite so encouraging, and I told him of my past experience with Tofranil.

'Don't worry, I'll try you on something different,' he assured me. 'Some of the side effects may be a bit unpleasant until you get used to them, but you must persevere, otherwise I cannot help you. The biggest mistake people make is stopping this type of medication before it has had a chance to work – and it does take a few weeks.'

He advised me of some of the usual side effects – dry mouth, drowsiness, constipation and blurred vision, which did not sound too great a menu to me. He also explained that antidepressants don't actually cure the depression – they just control it by working on the brain. The depression must run its course, and it would take time.

I froze. So there was no actual cure for this condition – it just continued until it was ready to stop. 'What's the longest I can expect?' I asked, hoping my fear wasn't showing.

He told me that it varies from person to person, and there is no way of telling, but that one woman's depression lasted on and off for two years. 'That is not to say that yours will last anywhere near that long, of course,' he added.

I decided that he was being honest at least, because two years was indeed a long time to be depressed, but I did not like what I was reading between the lines.

'Why me?' The bewilderment must have been evident in my voice.

'Why not you?' he replied in a matter-of-fact tone. 'Some people develop heart disease, some cancer, some a disorder that affects the brain. It's an illness like any other. So why not you?'

I will never forget those words, which I have passed on to other people since, people who have asked me that same question. But at that time, all I could think of was the stigma attached to mental illness. If I had heart disease or cancer at least I could talk about it with other people, but mental illness was something that had to be hidden. I would have to carry on more or less alone.

How would I tell my family? It was a far cry from the brush with cancer, or ovarian cysts, when I was able to go home and say I needed surgery, knowing that everyone would be understanding, that it would all be over in a short space of time. How does one go home and say 'Guess what! I'm suffering from a mental illness and it could take many months to run its course!'? The family had already had enough of me and my panic attacks. They most certainly did not need any further shocks. And would they believe me anyway? If I, understanding and tolerant by nature, found it difficult to believe, I could hardly expect them to accept it readily.

Dr W. broke in on my thoughts at this point, telling me I was to stop the Serepax completely. He was not happy that I was using it, particularly in such large quantities. He would wean me off it by using a small dose of diazepam (Valium) in its place, and then wean me off the Valium which is much easier to discontinue.

He talked on reassuringly for a while, but I found it difficult to concentrate on what he was saying. He eventually ushered me out, again shaking my hand in a warm, comforting manner. But this time I took no comfort from this man who had not only dashed all my hopes, but labelled me mentally ill.

I felt wounded and crushed as I left his office armed with prescriptions for Valium and the antidepressant Sinequan, still trying to digest all I had just been told. I had gone through my whole life not knowing that there was such a thing as endogenous depression. It was bizarre that I should now be affected by it. Diabetes would have been a much more civilised affliction had I had the choice. That was also in the family history.

I puffed on a cigarette as I sat in the car in the parking lot for what seemed an eternity, not wanting to go home, not knowing how I would break the news to my family. The word 'endogenous' kept rolling over and over in my mind, with pictures of out-of-balance chemicals floating around in my head. How on earth would I cope with the side effects of antidepressants and still go to work? How depressed could I expect to be – down in the dumps, awfully miserable, or very very unhappy? I simply could not imagine being very unhappy for any length of time, particularly without an obvious reason. I just didn't see myself as a weepy, depressed person. Bizarre scenes from *One Flew Over the Cuckoo's Nest* wafted into my mind. I had never had any contact with mental illness, although during panic attacks in the car I had often visualised myself losing control of my sanity and 'flipping out' completely. Was this also likely to happen to me? I should have thought to ask!

I eventually started the car, still deep in thought, and made my way home in a sort of nervous trance. I would probably just blurt it out to the family, because no matter how I phrased it they would all say 'Rubbish! You've got nothing to be depressed about.' George's family would not take too kindly to mental illness, and they would not believe the word of a psychiatrist – in their eyes a 'quack' or drug-pusher. Even my own family would warn me against seeing a psychiatrist.

George and his family reacted exactly as I thought they would. I tried explaining that frightening word 'endogenous', but that was of no help either. There are not too many families who would react calmly to such a bolt of lightning in their lives. But it saddened and frightened me that I would have to cope alone not only with the illness and the medication, but also with the attitudes of those around me. Ahead I could see an up-hill battle on a lonely road. I could only hope it would not be too long.

I did not know then that it would take four long years before some members of both families would accept my condition for what it was. The general cry was 'Change of life, my dear'. It hurt deeply that they did not believe me and left me no support other than my doctor.

Many people, particularly in the older generation, have no concept of mental illness in any form. Talking to one such woman some time ago and knowing there had been a lot of 'nervous' disorders in her family, I asked her if there had been any actual mental illness in the family. Her immediate response was 'no', but when we touched on the question of suicide she mentioned that an aunt had committed suicide, although she was unable to relate it to depression or mental illness in any way. She simply did not understand the real meaning of depression at all.

Understanding depression

We all understand the meaning of unhappiness and sadness, and we hear the words 'I'm depressed' so often that we assume we know the meaning of depression also. But do we?

There is a vast difference between sadness and depression, and only those who have experienced both can really understand what that difference is. True clinical depression is not merely the 'blues', or even the normal sadness that accompanies loss. It is a devastating and debilitating illness that lasts for many months if left untreated. It is also the most common and the most life-threatening of the serious mental illnesses. Many of the suicides and attempted suicides that take place are the result of depression, so we must be thankful that it is also one of the more easily treated mental illnesses.

Let us look at a few examples of unhappiness and depression.

Jenny's date has just rung to say they will have to skip the movie they had planned for tonight because he has to work late. Jenny has been looking forward to this movie all week, she's excited, and is dressed and ready to go. How could he do this to her? She slams the phone down and throws herself on the bed. Her night is ruined and she feels miserable and depressed. But is she? No, although she would no doubt say she was, if asked. Her feelings would probably be disappointment, anger and frustration, and those feelings would soon fly out the window if her date rang back to say they could go to the movies after all.

Margaret is suffering premenstrual tension, when she always feels angry and dejected, and things generally go wrong for her. Today has been a particularly bad day, and she has ended up feeling thoroughly miserable. This 'downer' is very real for Margaret, but is only temporary. She knows that; knows too that a call from an understanding friend, or an unexpected pleasant surprise, would lift her mood somewhat.

Julie is crying in her husband's arms, seeking comfort because her father died recently. She feels a very real sadness that no phone call or pleasant surprise can lift. But her sadness is a natural response to a very sad loss, and in the natural passage of time her grief will run its course and she will return to normal mood.

Then we look at Jack. At six in the evening he is still at the office, slumped in his chair, staring out of the window at the overcast sky which truly reflects his feelings. There is a heaviness in his body, and it is too much of an effort to get out of his chair and prepare for the drive home. He has had a lousy day, unable to concentrate on his work, and has made mistakes that normally he would never make. He now feels that he is letting everybody down. He has no interest in eating, or anything else for that matter. He does not sleep well, does not have any interest in his wife any more, and his sex drive has completely disappeared. Jack has been in this mood, for no apparent reason, for some weeks now and no amount of coaxing or concern from his wife, family or friends has been able to penetrate his wall of gloom. Jack is truly depressed.

So we can see the difference between unhappiness, sadness and depression. When we are sad, we are experiencing a normal reaction to loss or pain, and no matter how great the loss or pain, we will eventually be able to accept the comfort of those who reach out to us, to be kind to ourselves. We know that the distressing emotions will pass. But if we are truly depressed, we are isolated from the rest of the world behind a thick impenetrable wall. The disturbance of mood in the psychotic depressive state is qualitatively different from normal everyday depression. It has a numbing effect on the whole person, it arises inexplicably, and it is of a depth and type that cannot be alleviated by the usual measures of comfort offered.

Others offer concern, but they are unable to reach us – and we have lost the capacity to reach out to them, or even to be kind to ourselves. We no longer experience the ebb and flow of normal emotions. We have completely lost the spirit of life, and are filled with a horrible sense of emptiness.

Following any major setback in our lives it is usual for us to experience a period of sadness, withdrawal, anxiety and sleep disturbance, but we soon re-establish our normal mood and get on with our lives. When a depression persists, however, and the person develops the symptoms that Jack has displayed, and those symptoms are ongoing at that level for some weeks, he is said to be suffering a clinical depression. That is, the mood has shifted from what is considered normal, to a *medical condition*, and the process may not necessarily have been set off by any event in his life such as failure, disillusionment or loss.

If we were now to go back to the beginning of Jack's depression, we would see that he is no longer able to derive any *interest or pleasure* from activities he used to enjoy. His mates might coax him into a game of golf and a few drinks, but he would just be going through the motions for their sakes. And his wife would be searching his eyes for a spark of the life they once held, wondering what had happened to the Jack she used to know.

Jack could now spiral down into an even deeper depression where he sees the world around him as if through a fog, drained of colour, and his inner world becomes black. Due to visual disturbances that take place, it is common for people in the throes of major depression to perceive the world around them as being a long way away, often shrouded in fog, and for colours to appear drab and grey. They cannot see clearly what lies beyond a certain distance from where they stand. Their inner world becomes dark and distorted, and they see no light at the end of the tunnel.

In *Depression and How to Survive It* by Spike Milligan and Dr Anthony Clare, Spike Milligan was asked, 'Why is it so difficult to describe?' He replied:

> It's invisible. There's no written diagrams. It's an abstract, it's a sensation, and if you ask people to paint it most depressives will draw black. Have you noticed that? Black paintings all over the place, so we know it has no colour for a start.

When asked to describe it at a later date whilst in the grip of severe depression, Spike said:

> There is this terrible emptiness. I just want to go away, disappear, cover myself up until it goes away. It is like pain yet it is not a physical pain. I cannot describe it. It is like every fibre in your body is screaming for relief yet there is no relief. How can I describe it? I cannot really. I cannot, of course, escape because I have to keep working, which I just about do – though once

or twice I have had to stop, had to just hide away and wait till I could summon up the energy just to keep going.

At this point Dr Clare noted that Spike, normally fast and furious with words, had to make a Herculean effort just to make conversation. Responding to questions about how he felt took an almost physical struggle. Spike also referred to the black void so often experienced by depressed people: '…The whole world is taken away, all there is is this black void, this terrible, terrible, empty, aching, black void …'

That black void is what Jack would now be experiencing. He has been stripped of the ability to experience normal emotions, no longer even able to love or accept the love of others. Alone in his dark world, he is filled with the horror of his emptiness. One by one his emotions have all been drained away – happiness, affection, humour and pride. All gone. He knows there was a time when he had been able to experience these emotions, but no matter how hard he tries, he can no longer remember how it felt to love and be loved, to enjoy a good laugh, or even a good meal. He is experiencing the death of his spirit, known in psychiatric terms as anhedonia.

Dr Clare sums up the usual symptoms of depression in the seriously depressed:

Seriously depressed individuals describe an overall deadening of sensation. Food becomes bland, dry, tasteless. Sound becomes either distant or horrendously loud and intrusive. For Milligan, the merest sound when he is depressed can render him immobile with pain. Colour, as he observes above, drains from the environment – grey-black predominates. Smell fades. Touch dulls. The emotions drain away such that the truly depressed fear they have lost the power to respond to concern, affection, love with any human feeling whatever.

We endure persecution
but we are not forsaken;
we are cast down,
but we do not perish.

2 Corinthians 4:9

4 After diagnosis

Like Jack, I had been suffering from most of the usual symptoms of depression for some time, without realising what was happening to me. It was with some trepidation that I started on my Sinequan capsules as prescribed by Dr W. The effects, although not as severe as those caused by the Tofranil, were nonetheless unpleasant. I was dizzy as I got out of bed, and had to be careful to stand up very slowly. My mouth was constantly parched and I seemed to be drinking gallons of liquid every day. The biggest problem, however, was staying awake at work because of extreme drowsiness, but I still had to carry on with my daily life. I wondered how I would manage as the dosage was increased to the maximum level.

Friends at work were marvellous. Once they discovered I had a problem, and had consulted a psychiatrist, they were most supportive. I discovered to my amazement that several people related to my situation.

Jacqui came up to me during one morning tea break. 'I'm glad you did the right thing and went to a psychiatrist,' she said. 'I *thought* you were depressed.'

I was floored, and even more so to find out she had actually taken Sinequan herself. 'Yes. The side effects are a bit uncomfortable at first,' she said, 'but don't give up, because eventually they'll help you. Sinequan is very good.'

I don't think she'll ever know what a comfort she was when I needed it most. When I was expecting to be labelled 'crazy', I found people who understood — understood to a degree, that is. I soon discovered that people shied away from the word 'endogenous', believing that emotional problems were causing my depression. They could not accept the very real diagnosis of mental illness. Eventually I too found myself doubting the doctor's diagnosis because I did not want to accept the stigma of being 'different'.

Time and time again as I turned everything over in my mind, I knew I should have faith in my doctor's diagnosis, but a part of me kept grasping at the more tangible things in my life as a possible cause. Being depressed, my mind turned easily to all the unhappy events in my life and magnified them a thousand times. Soon it was much easier to say the depression was caused by lack of emotional fulfilment in my marriage, or problems in childhood or adolescence. And I began to believe it. After all, it was much more acceptable than the stigma of endogenous depression.

Tim Finn, singer and songwriter, formerly of Split Enz, talked of the difficulties of admitting to depression (Janet Hawley, 'The Darkness Within', *Good Weekend*, 29 April 1995):

> There's something taboo about admitting you're depressed, which is terrible. It would be a wonderful freedom for people if they were taught – around these ages, or those situations – you'll probably become depressed, and it's okay, go into it, learn from it.

Tim has learned from his depression – he says that a lot of symbols and images come from life's most bleak moments, that his best songs come from periods when he is just moving out of deep sorrow.

On the other side of the coin, Sydney psychiatrist Dr Morison Tarrant talked in the same article of the pain of his crippling depression, saying it was:

> … unrelenting agony. I'll never forget it however long I live and just talking about it fills me with fear. I don't want to go back there … People say to me 'Oh you've had this profound experience, you must have got a lot of personal growth out of it'… I haven't learned shit, okay … Depression is a waste of time that could have been lived. And you didn't just waste it, you spent it in agony.

We may not be able to ease the pain of depression, but it would certainly help our ultimate progress to be shown the same acceptance and respect as the person with a physical illness. In the long term, however, like Tim I now believe that we can learn from our illness, even though our everyday lives are more difficult to contend with than when we were well and even though the illness may remain with us to varying degrees for the rest of our lives. We can ultimately learn much about ourselves and others, learn to change our priorities in life and have different perspectives on many areas of life, culture and society – all of which can have a very positive effect.

Back in my early periods of deep depression, however, it was not so easy for me, with nobody believing in my doctor's diagnosis, nobody to truly support me as a person with a mental illness. I threw suggestions of emotional illness to Dr W., which he very deftly threw back to me. He listened, as he always did, to everything I had to say, discussed it with me, then told me that these were separate issues, nothing to do with the onset of my depression. 'We will deal with all these things when you're well,' he said.

As I continued sinking into a deeper depression, I was scared because life as I had always known it was slipping away from me and I was out of control. It seemed that I was a completely different person on the inside with no visible signs on the outside to help people understand what was happening to me. I had lost all interest in myself, my friends, even my family, and yet I had to continue working and smiling, showing the world that I was normal. It was a bizarre and frightening situation.

Many people initially visit their doctor because of one of the physical symptoms of depression such as insomnia, early morning awakenings, loss of energy, constipation, poor appetite, tiredness and loss of libido. But these symptoms do not describe the human feelings. The people who responded to my questionnaire talked, among other things, of low self-esteem and feelings of failure, constant negative thinking contrary to their usual nature, guilt feelings, the hopelessness that arises from being unable to see an end to their plight, the pain of thinking that their family did not love them, and of not being able to participate in normal everyday life. And of course there were the pervasive self-destructive thoughts.

As the mood departs from normal and starts its downward spiral, certain changes take place and continue to do so, like links in a never-ending chain. One of the first is the change in sleeping patterns. It could be trouble going to sleep, waking during the night and being unable to go back to sleep, or it could be the dreaded early-morning awakenings around four o'clock. These are typically accompanied by acute anxiety, self-accusations and searing guilt feelings that cannot be quelled. Minor misdeeds going back as far as childhood are blown up out of all proportion, and the accompanying guilt is excessive, leaving the person writhing in shame and torment.

That is how it was with me. I became tired and even more anxious, my agoraphobia now completely out of hand, so it was not long before I was again taking Mogadon at night to give me sufficient sleep to get through the following day at work.

Constipation was another big problem. It would often be ten days to two weeks before I realised that I was very bloated. There were times when I had spasms of the colon and was often immobilised on the bathroom floor by waves of intense pain, rising and falling, reminiscent of labour pains.

I seemed always to be in turmoil, a mixture of panic attacks and depression, with Dr W. steadfastly telling me one thing, my friends convinced he was wrong, and me wanting to believe them, not him. No matter how much I trusted him, I did not want to be mentally ill.

And then there was George, whose whole world had fallen apart as he watched his wife taking drugs but still slipping further and further into depression. He quite naturally blamed the drugs for my tiredness and lack of communication, and was not in any frame of mind to discuss the illness calmly with my doctor. Our many arguments were causing a huge rift in our relationship and, as the rift widened, I began to blame him for my state of mind, each argument being magnified out of all proportion by my depression.

Natalie was in Year 11 at school and going through her own teenage traumas at the time, and Tanya was at the vulnerable age of fourteen. In the past I had always been there for them in every way, but now, little by little, I was being taken away just when they needed me most.

Yes, the winter of 1988 was a particularly bleak one. Not only did I have to cope with the usual daily tasks at home and at work, but I was also plagued with confusion, embarrassment, guilt and humiliation. Plagued, too, with the deepening depression, the constant panic attacks and the still seemingly impossible task of coming off Serepax. I remember one particularly embarrassing panic attack in our local supermarket, one of the many that had resulted in my developing agoraphobia. The following is quoted directly from my journal, giving you an idea of the fear I experienced during those attacks:

> Everything seemed to be fading away before my eyes and the floor was spinning away from beneath my feet, leaving a huge gaping black hole. I couldn't see properly. My heart was thumping and racing, I was shaking uncontrollably, and beads of perspiration covered my entire face. What a mess I must have looked. I felt myself teetering, and thought I was going to

fall into a void. I clutched the trolley as I dropped down to the floor. I huddled up, kneeling close to the shelves with my head on my knees, trying to shut it all out. Please, God, help me. I was close to blacking out, absolutely terrified. I thought my heart would stop, or at the very least, burst. My head was like a balloon just waiting for someone to stick the pin in.

I'm trapped! Can't breathe. Can't just leave the trolley and try and make it to the door. I wouldn't make it anyway. I'd collapse in a heap. Why is everything fading away? Why do people look distorted? My God, what if I look as bad as I feel! I can't let people know I'm out of control. I've got to stand up, pretend nothing's wrong. But I'll have to go now, I can't finish the shopping.

I tried to collect my thoughts. What if I did black out? What would happen? What would people think? And if I didn't, how would I finish my shopping? How would my legs support me? Could I stand in the queue at the checkout? Would I 'flip out' in front of the cashier? Or would I panic, leave my trolley with her, and race outside? But then I'd really look odd. People would know there was something wrong with me. No, I must look calm. Could I drive home? I wasn't safe on the roads. Would I make it? I want to go home, to lie down, to sleep. I don't want to flip out here.

As these terrifying scenes flashed through my mind, I did what I knew I had to, to survive. I took a Valium.

A voice broke through my fear. 'Are you all right?'

I don't know how I answered or what I said, but I mumbled something about being OK, feeling terribly embarrassed. I just wanted to lie down, to wait for it to subside.

I managed to finish my shopping that day as I always did, but I was in a daze that prevented my making good decisions. I just wanted to get out of that dreadful situation and home to my couch. Rest was the only thing that ever helped me.

I discovered that depression makes it difficult to relate to other people, and because of the agoraphobia I shied away from making social engagements that I knew I would ultimately break due to fear. So I went to great lengths to avoid people, avoid being drawn into conversation. I watched from the sidelines as my friends enjoyed their lives and I envied their happiness, their ability to be normal. I'd have loved to join in, but fear and lack of energy and interest held me back.

I realised eventually that Dr W. was right about the Sinequan. With perseverence, there was a noticeable improvement over the next few months. But not enough. So he added Lithium to my menu of daily pills. Here was yet another curve ball for me to deal with, because I had associated Lithium with people in mental institutions. But I was getting much better at accepting new and unpleasant things, and handled this one quite well.

One week later Dr W. ordered routine blood tests to determine the level of Lithium in my blood, and the results showed up yet another surprise. I had an underactive thyroid gland. This was very interesting, because depression can be a symptom of an underactive thyroid gland, and he hoped that there would be some improvement in my condition once the thyroid problem was treated. This was the first real glimmer of hope for me as I started taking Oroxine, a thyroid medication.

There was no marked difference. To make matters worse, I had started putting on lots of weight. My appetite was now enormous, and the more I grew, the more I hated myself, and the more I ate to console myself. It was a very vicious circle. Cream cakes had become my big outlet. There was a wonderful cake shop in Carlisle Street and I was drawn to it like a magnet every day, buying two or three cakes each time, eating them all in one sitting, usually in the car park by the shopping centre. At times I bought extras to eat in the car on the way home.

I started buying 'fat' clothes to hide the weight, and the person in the mirror was suddenly not the person I knew, but some loathsome, undisciplined blob. 'Don't worry,' friends said. 'It always happens when you're depressed.' But words didn't help. I hated myself, hated the fatness, hated the lack of self-control.

Dr W. had warned me that Sinequan could cause a weight gain, but this was quite ridiculous. As fast as I grew into my new fat clothes, I grew out of them again. It was humiliating. I had become a compulsive eater with a driving need to quell the withdrawal symptoms, to satisfy the never-ending obsession that gnawed at me.

Once the binge was over, I would be filled with a deep sense of peace and contentment. But only for a while. Waves of guilt and shame soon followed. Everyone else looked slim. I saw nothing but perfect people with perfect bodies, and I envied their self-control, acutely aware that mine had completely deserted me. I squirmed and cringed, despising the gluttonous creature I'd become. At that moment, if food was available, I would eat again to dispel the depressive feelings.

Eating soon became a daily ritual, my comfort zone. Obviously it had a lot to do with quelling all my inner turmoil – the anxiety, depression and low self-esteem, – but I was blinded by the firm belief that it was only the antidepressant medication causing the increased appetite. I knew that one day I would be telling Dr W. that I wanted to stop taking them.

Tis the human touch in this world that counts,
The touch of your hand and mine,
Which means far more to the fainting heart
Than shelter and bread and wine ...

Spencer Michael Free

5 Anxiety, panic and phobic disorders

Anxiety

Anxiety is that 'sinking in the stomach' feeling, often accompanied by beads of perspiration across the forehead, or sweaty palms, which we have all experienced when we thought that something unpleasant was going to happen. Most of us describe anxiety by saying we're 'apprehensive', 'uptight', 'on edge', or 'keyed up' about some anticipated happening. It is our response to what we see as a threat.

A certain amount of anxiety is a normal part of life. It reaches into our work environment, social affairs and home life, and is often responsible for the dark circles under our eyes after a sleepless night. It affects everyone, from those on the assembly line to top-line executives. No one is immune, although usually women tend to feel more anxious more often, and over more things, than men. I remember saying of my mother that if life were going perfectly smoothly for all of us she would worry about the fact that there was nothing to worry about.

In today's society there are many who are fearful of losing their livelihood, there are relationships that are unstable or have broken down, and there are concerns about the changing roles of both men and women.

Parents worry about their children. Are they as happy and well-adjusted as they should be? As a parent am I doing what is necessary to ensure that they are? As well, every day our living rooms are invaded by local and world issues on radio and TV, most of which we are powerless to deal with.

There are also the more abstract threats, however, that relate to our self-esteem and confidence. Children feel apprehensive if other children don't like them, and some are almost constantly anxious about being unable to satisfy the high expectations of their parents. Even though many of those insecurities and anxieties are left behind with childhood, we still retain one basic need, to be liked and loved – the 'human touch' of which Spencer Michael Free writes, from which stem a lot of our intangible anxieties. And there are those individuals who, despite being liked and loved, are continually plagued by doubts of their own self-worth.

Normal anxiety is related to something specific such as exam results or a visit to the dentist, and it has a limited life. Once the cause has passed, the anxiety also disappears. If we look at it in the context of a response to a threat, anxiety can sometimes be used to advantage, to enhance performance. Students' anxiety before an exam, for example, might make them strive harder, and ultimately give them a great sense of satisfaction when they achieve a mark higher than expected. And how often does our anxiety spur us on to make decisions, take positive steps to find solutions to our problems? Actors and musicians have often said they need that rush of adrenaline before each performance.

To better understand anxiety we need to recognise the ways in which our bodies react to a threat or fear. There is both a physical and a mental response, the physical signs being related to the 'fight or flight' instinct, without which our prehistoric ancestors would not have survived. This response is triggered by the sympathetic nervous system, which stimulates a discharge of the stress hormones adrenaline and noradrenaline from the adrenal glands. These hormones prime the body for action by increasing heart rate, breathing, alertness and muscle response, and virtually shutting down the digestive system. Thus we feel our heart thumping, our muscles tensed, and our breathing becoming more rapid.

In this aroused state, the mind also becomes more active and watchful and, if there is no obvious external threat, it searches for the reason for its distress, and over-reacts to everyday occurrences. Thus the anxious person often cannot sit still, fidgets, and is so tense with fearful anticipation that even the opening of a door will startle her or him.

These days, although we no longer have to contend with wild animals, we still need our inherent fear mechanism. Should a burglar enter our home, for instance, our bodies would react in the same way, preparing us for fight or flight, releasing the energy for us to leap into action. Of course, many of the threats to our well-being are more intangible, where the fight-or-flight response is neither needed nor useful. Our bodies are in a heightened state, showing all the fight or flight signs, with no way of releasing the pent-up energy. So we carry it with us, perhaps for the whole day, perhaps even to bed. The results can be physically and psychologically harmful if we allow these reactions to continue without finding alternative methods of coping with our anxieties.

Worse still, the symptoms of severe anxiety can appear for no apparent external reason, causing extreme panic.

Anxiety state

Many people suffer from seemingly inexplicable attacks of anxiety from time to time when there is no obvious threat in their lives. Research shows that thirty to forty per cent of the general population have sufficiently high levels of anxiety to benefit from professional help. The symptoms of these attacks are much more intense and painful than usual, come swiftly and unexpectedly, and are all the more terrifying because there is no apparent cause. Between 'attacks', these people will probably have levels of anxiety much higher than is normal. When a person is unable to cope effectively with the demands of daily life due to apprehension and tensions, the condition must be regarded as a psychiatric disorder, which requires treatment and care.

The registering of emotions in such a person has become exaggerated to the point where an ordinary flash of fear or anxiety becomes a flash of panic (a 'panic attack'), often having the effect of an electric shock. Panic is a sudden and excessive feeling of fright that strikes us when we feel we cannot deal successfully with a situation. We panic when we lack confidence in our reactions to given circumstances; we fear losing control. The key to whether we become completely immobilised is the length of time we are in a state of panic, and how often it occurs. People in this state usually think either that there is something physically wrong or that they are going crazy.

The first instinct will be to flee, to get as far away as possible, or to head for fresh air and then the car, to try to regain composure. The mind searches for a reason for the panic – there has to be a reason. If there is no external reason perhaps the individual will decide to slow down a bit or eat better meals, and see the whole episode in terms of its being ridiculous.

The mind, however, does not so easily let go of such an experience when there is no suitable explanation. Unfortunately, the more attention given to the fear, the more fear is experienced and the more the panic attacks strike. It becomes a vicious cycle that is difficult to break without help. One soon feels totally under the control of some mysterious 'thing' that has taken over one's life without reason.

Every strategy is used in the determination to beat it: sheer willpower, hypnotherapy, relaxation tapes, and so on. But nothing works and, indeed, the more attention is focused on it, the more it continues to dominate one's life. The ability to relax is lost, either alone or in others' company; day-to-day work and social life is interfered with; and the ability to have happy and positive thoughts about what the future may hold is denied one. It is so pervasive, in fact, that no area of life is spared.

Such a person is said to be in an 'anxiety state', suffering from 'free-floating anxiety' or 'generalised anxiety disorder'.

Many people think that stress and anxiety are the same, but this is not so. Stress equates to pressure, and stress occurs when pressure is applied from an outside source. Anxiety, on the other hand, arises from within the person. It should be noted, however, that there is a relationship between the two, in that severe anxiety will cause the sufferer to be highly stressed by the mere fact of having to contend with it on a day-to-day basis. By the same token, when the demands of life become excessive, this places stress upon us, and those who are perhaps genetically more vulnerable to anxiety will see these demands as a threat, and will display anxiety symptoms.

It would be wise, then, for anxiety sufferers to restrict their stress load as much as possible in all areas of their lives, to ensure they obtain sufficient sleep, and to follow a healthy diet and exercise program. We all know that long-term stress can be serious in that it affects the blood vessels, and is linked with heart attacks, skin complaints, and a suppressed immune system that can make us more susceptible to infections and even to cancer.

Anxiety and depression often go hand-in-hand, although we do not consciously connect the two. A mother, for example, could be very anxious sitting in the doctor's waiting room with her sick child, and if the child is then hospitalised for a period, no one will be surprised to see the mother show signs of depression. This exemplifies the normal ebb and flow of emotions, of course, and once the child is well again, the mother's anxiety and depression will quickly lift. Similarly, we find that an anxiety state often goes hand-in-hand with clinical depression but, unfortunately, the clinical depression makes treatment of the anxiety state much more difficult.

From my reading, it seems that women suffer from severe anxiety more than men; it affects people from all social, economic and education levels; and more often than not it affects people whose lives are busy and productive. They are usually obliging people, eager to please, to be positive, and not to criticise others. But they also have low self-esteem, often feel left out, and are always looking to accept blame.

Phobias

Phobias are related to anxiety but, rather than being abstract fears, or fears about future events, they focus on some specific object or situation, which a person knows to be irrational and out of all proportion to the circumstances, but which simply cannot be controlled.

Most of us have at least one fear that we would prefer to conceal. It may be of spiders, snakes, heights, enclosed spaces, flying, or a variety of other things. Most of us accept our fears as normal, however, and put up with the anxiety they cause, or take steps to avoid what frighten us. It is when the fear becomes excessive and disrupts our lives that we call it a phobia.

For example, I have a spider phobia (arachnophobia), and if I see a spider I become almost paralysed with fear. It will have to be killed, although I cannot do it myself, and I will I be vigilant for weeks to come. I had a friend who was so frightened of birds (ornithophobia) that she lost control of her car when a bird flew in front of the windscreen. Her state of shock when she was taken to the hospital was more the result of seeing the bird than of the effects of the relatively minor accident. For people suffering from fear of enclosed spaces (claustrophobia), elevators, buses and planes can be a real nightmare. A fear of elevators may be so great that an individual would have a very real problem attending an appointment on the twelfth floor of a building, and might well decide to use the stairs.

Classification of some phobias

Phobia	Fear of
acrophobia	heights
aerophobia	draughts
agoraphobia	open spaces

aichmophobia	sharp objects
ailurophobia	cats
algophobia	pain
androphobia	men
anthophobia	flowers
anthropophobia	people
aquaphobia	water
astraphobia	lightning
bacteriophobia	bacteria
bathophobia	depth
brontophobia	thunder
claustrophobia	closed spaces
cynophobia	dogs
demonophobia	demons
dromophobia	crossing streets
equinophobia	horses
genophobia	sex
gynophobia	women
haptephobia	being touched
herpetophobia	creeping, crawling things
hypsophobia	falling
hypnophobia	going to sleep
mysophobia	dirt, germs, contamination
neophobia	anything new
numerophobia	numbers
nycotophobia	darkness
ochiophobia	crowds
pyrophobia	fire
scotophobia	blindness
taphophobia	being buried alive
theophobia	God
xenophobia	strangers
zoophobia	animals

(This table is taken from 'Panic and phobic disorders', Fiona K. Judd & Graham D. Burrows, *Australian Family Physician*, vol. 15, no. 2, February 1986, p. 152.)

Panic and phobic disorders

Years ago, anxiety was always referred to as nervousness, with some people suffering mild and acute bouts, others suffering severe chronic states. Today we still hear many people saying they suffer from 'nerves', although the disorder is now becoming more widely known among lay people as 'anxiety'. Similarly, panic disorder (as it is now termed) was once considered to be a form of recurring attacks of anxiety or nervousness. It was not until 1978 that separate diagnostic criteria were established for panic disorder, and not until 1980 that it was actually included in the American Psychiatric Association's Diagnostic and Statistical Manual (DSM III) for mental disorders.

Panic disorder seems to occur more frequently in women, and is very common. I think many of us have long since recognised this in many cultures, in many countries, even though we may not have given voice to our opinion. What is perhaps not so widely known is that it typically starts in late adolescence or early adulthood. We do not expect young people to suffer from this disorder. We expect them to be consumed by the passion for living a full life. But if we stop and think, we *do* hear young people complaining of feeling 'stressed out'; however, we often put it down to the hectic pace of modern-day living. Perhaps we should listen and observe more closely. It is *not* a state experienced exclusively by thirty- to forty-year-olds. In fact, it is rather unusual for panic attacks to commence after the age of forty.

After suffering a number of panic attacks in varying situations, many sufferers begin to anticipate further attacks in those same situations. This anticipation brings with it a great fear of the crippling effects already experienced. It is this secondary fear that brings about a phobia. The type of phobia depends on the situation in which the attacks previously occurred. Perhaps it was in an elevator; then claustrophobia sets in. Perhaps it was in open or public places; then agoraphobia is the result. The place or situation will then be avoided, although it is the panic attack rather than the place or situation that is really feared.

Eventually, when the condition becomes really disabling, people scurry off to their doctor hoping for a magic cure. If the person is quickly diagnosed and referred to a specialist in this field, appropriate treatment can bring relief, prevent the condition worsening, and prevent other medical conditions arising as a result of the stress placed on the body.

Slowly but surely, this will provide the sufferer with the skills necessary to confront, cope with, and eventually overcome the disorder.

In 'Panic and phobic disorders' (*Australian Family Physician*, vol. 15, no. 2, February 1986) Fiona K. Judd and Graham D. Burrows state that:

> Patients with panic disorder have twice the risk of hypertension and peptic ulcer as members of the general population. Male patients are more likely to die from resulting cardiovascular disease or suicide. Depression is common in these patients ... It has been estimated that five per cent to ten per cent of patients with phobic anxiety develop secondary alcohol and drug abuse.

Judd and Burrows go on to say that 'increasing evidence suggests panic disorder is a metabolic disorder with genetic vulnerability'.

Diagnostic criteria for panic disorder

Fiona K. Judd and Graham D. Burrows (in the abovementioned article) set out the following as the diagnostic criteria for panic disorder:

- At least three panic attacks within a three-week period in circumstances other than during marked physical exertion or in a life-threatening situation. The attacks are not precipitated only by exposure to a circumscribed phobic stimulus.
- Panic attacks are manifested by discrete periods of apprehension or fear and at least four of the following symptoms appear during each attack:
  - dyspnoea [difficult or laboured breathing]
  - palpitations
  - chest pain or discomfort
  - choking or smothering sensations
  - dizziness, vertigo or unsteady feelings
  - feelings of unreality
  - parasthesias (tingling in hands or feet)
  - sweating
  - faintness
  - trembling or shaking
  - fear of dying, going crazy, or doing something uncontrolled during an attack.
- Not due to a physical or other mental disorder, such as major depression, somatisation disorder or schizophrenia.

Agoraphobia

The most disabling phobia is agoraphobia, which is often part of an anxiety state. This word is derived from the Greek words *phobos* meaning 'fear', and *agora* meaning 'a place of assembly' or 'market-place'. It is, therefore, usually described as a 'fear of public places' or 'fear of open spaces'. It is also referred to as a 'fear of leaving home'. But it is a little more complicated than any of these descriptions suggest.

It could be more accurately defined as a condition where people suffer such incapacitating fear (attacks of anxiety or panic) whilst away from home, that they will eventually fear returning to the place where the attack was experienced, because the memory is so frightening and painful, and they are fearful of its happening again. They are, in fact, afraid of their fear and its symptoms. If the attacks have occurred in a number of places, or perhaps also in a car or a bus, very soon such people will feel panicky whenever they have to leave the safety of home, and the fear could eventually keep them bound to the house, which is quite often what happens to agoraphobic individuals. At all costs, the distressing and painful attacks must be avoided.

But the degree to which the lives of these people are affected varies from one person to another. Some are happy to leave home as long as they are in the company of another person, while others cannot venture beyond the front door under any circumstances. Some are able to drive their car within certain known boundaries but will not venture into new areas, while others cannot drive at all without feeling unsafe. Some can drive their car but not walk down the street, while others have the opposite problem.

If you have not experienced a panic attack you will be unable to understand such intense and seemingly irrational fear. But you would understand if a friend involved in a serious car accident refused to drive a car again. The sudden impact and the realisation that they might not have survived the accident cause shock and acute anxiety, and the memory is so vivid and painful that they will avoid exposure to that kind of situation again. When this happens, we understand because there is a visible reason. But the fear and pain associated with a panic attack in an agoraphobic person are just as severe, just as real; it is only the cause that is different.

Such a person will probably be unable to explain, except to speak of the fear of fainting or collapsing in public and perhaps looking foolish.

The fear is actually of losing control when an attack takes hold, of being trapped, unable to make a quick escape from the terrifying situation, and perhaps to be unable to get help quickly in the event of losing control of the mind and of bodily functions.

Imagine the businesswoman about to address the directors at a board meeting, when suddenly she experiences the symptoms described on page 15. She panics, terrified at the prospect of having to deliver a speech in this condition. She is terrified of losing all control of her actions and rationality, of collapsing and making an exhibition of herself. She feels trapped! She will deliver her speech of course, despite her symptoms, but from then on the mere thought of walking into a board meeting could be enough to trigger a severe attack. Whilst anxiety during public speaking is now generally classified as a localised social phobia, the social phobia may co-exist in agoraphobia, and if that same woman has experienced these attacks in the supermarket, she will eventually fear the weekly shopping trips, attacks in the car will make it difficult to get to work which will be an enormous burden, and attacks in the street will restrict all areas of her life. This woman will probably struggle on with her life, albeit in a restricted manner, because she has no choice – she has to work – but she will eventually have to seek help to overcome the problem. The housewife, on the other hand, finding herself in the same panicky situations on a regular basis, is more likely to retreat to the safety of her home and stay there, perhaps venturing out only when she is with a family member or friend, because she does not have the same responsibilities in the outside world forcing her to carry on.

The agoraphobe fears situations in which he feels there is no way of escape. Therefore, if he *does* go to the cinema, a restaurant or church, he will make sure he has an aisle seat close to the door. If through necessity he travels on a bus, again he will sit or stand near the door, and if he is asked to move to the back of the bus, he might actually alight before his destination to avoid a distressing situation. The mass of people in a crowded department store might prevent him making a quick exit to the street. He feels claustrophobic. Eventually his whole life is fraught with fear.

Another common symptom of agoraphobia, a feeling of unreality, often occurs in busy streets or stores, but can happen anywhere. Surroundings and other people are seen as in an illusion or a dream, and the resulting feeling of disorientation can be very frightening. Some people find that wide streets or the vastness of an open highway and its surroundings produce this feeling, while in others the confines of a narrow street could be equally distressing.

Once the incapacitating fear has taken hold and the person retreats from life, relationships become very strained. One partner may not really understand the other's problem, and the preoccupation with the struggle to 'get through the day' leaves little energy or interest to accommodate the needs of others. They are no longer able to share the little pleasures of life – even a trip to the cinema becomes a painful and exhausting ordeal. So there is a great deal of misery and shame, not only for the sufferer, but for the family as well.

There is a great comedy called *What About Bob?*, which I would recommend to every anxious or phobic person. Poor Bob, frightened of everything in life, has been referred to a specialist about his fears. On arrival at the doctor's address he discovers that the doctor's suite is on the forty-fourth floor. After a moment of panic his more rational side takes over and he approaches the elevator. He takes only a few faltering steps, however, before backing off and climbing the stairs, and arrives, exhausted, at his doctor's door. But by the time the consultation is over, he has gained some confidence and decides to take the elevator down. Courageous Bob! The elevator has not travelled very far when Bob's fears return, and his loud, terrified scream precedes him down the elevator shaft to the ground floor.

Like most sufferers of anxiety and agoraphobia, Bob is prone to hyperventilating, and in another scene he is shown breathing into his trusty paper bag on a crowded bus, trying desperately to gain some relief. The person who constantly hyperventilates never goes anywhere without that little paper bag.

You can be helped

Fortunately, there is help available for sufferers of severe anxiety, agoraphobia and other phobias, although the methods do require courage and hard work on the part of the sufferer. There is no 'magic pill' that will provide an instant cure, and no one who can 'cure' the sufferer without that person's help.

Obviously the first step is to identify your problem and then to acquire as much knowledge about the condition as possible. There are a number of excellent books available that not only explain what is happening to you, but also detail ways of facing and overcoming your fears. Most people approach their doctor for help, and if this is your first course of action you should discuss with her or him the various types of treatment available. You may be prescribed tranquillisers initially, but you could also be recommended another form of treatment, and you may be referred to a therapist or psychologist.

Some will respond to one or more of the methods mentioned in the chapter on treatments but, because of the very nature of this illness, many agoraphobes will find it difficult to leave the safety of their home for the necessary visits to their therapist. Self-help books and tapes available from the local library may help in this regard, as can telephone counselling services.

One thing is certain – you *can* overcome your fear. It will take longer and be more difficult if you also suffer from depression or manic-depression, but even if such complications do exist, you can exert a large measure of control over your anxiety if you are prepared to be patient and tolerant whilst confronting your fears. But *you* must be the one to make the first move, to seek help. Agoraphobes tend not to accept their fears, battling on with fierce determination to overcome their problems alone. It was that way with me in 1987 when I was first overcome by anxiety, but eventually I had no choice.

I walk through the shadow of death,
I will fear no evil:
For Thou art with me;
Thy rod and Thy staff they comfort me.

Psalm 23

6 Characteristics of manic-depressive illness

About the illness

By the time I had begun to comprehend the true meaning of my depression and agoraphobia, there came the even more bizarre symptoms of hypomania. The depression seemed rather like being thrown off a cliff into a bottomless pit with weights tied to my feet, being transported down to the depths of a dark world where I did not belong and from which there was no return, and whilst the manic episodes were either the most exciting times of my life or the most frenzied and bizarre, they were always soul-destroying.

And it all happened so suddenly, being transported from the world of normal existence to the alien world of mental illness.

I discovered that the person suffering from the disorder known as manic-depressive illness (also called 'manic-depressive psychosis') will experience 'highs' (periods of reckless elation, increased rate of thinking, hyperactivity and supreme confidence) called mania or hypomania, as well as 'lows' (periods of morbid despair, loss of interest, guilt, and a slowing of mental and physical functioning) called major or 'psychotic' depression, with relatively normal periods in between. Psychiatrists now refer to this as bipolar disorder, so named because the mood swings oscillate between the two poles of reckless ecstasy and morbid despair. A person suffering out-and-out manic episodes as well as some periods of depression is said to have Bipolar I disorder, and the person suffering hypomanic episodes (a more controlled state of mania) as well as severe depression is said to have Bipolar II disorder. Those suffering recurrent severe depression without the highs are said to have unipolar major depression, and those suffering only the manic highs with little or no depression are said to have unipolar mania, which is extremely rare.

These mood disorders are called major affective disorders – 'affective' being the word traditionally used by psychologists and philosophers for emotion or one's spirits.

While the experts agree that there are some psychological components to manic-depressive illness, it is viewed today primarily as a medical disorder resulting from abnormal brain chemistry – a disorder that affects mood, thinking and behaviour, the treatment of which rests firmly in the realms of both medicine and psychology.

Typically, episodes of these illnesses are time-limited. They come and go, last from several weeks to several months and are followed by periods of relatively normal mood and behaviour. Left untreated, however, the episodes will be longer – an episode of depression can last twelve months or more without remission.

Obviously then, it is crucial that treatment be sought immediately the problem is recognised. The unfortunate part is that, with a first episode, the person does not realise what is happening to her: she is confused, unable to explain it to those around her, who are also confused and often angered by her unusual and annoying behaviour; and so treatment is often delayed. What they do not realise is that these illnesses are powerful and insidious, and once they take hold the person is without the power to lighten or temper her mood or symptoms. Quite simply, she has lost control of the state of her mind.

In an instant a person can be lifted by this illness from the limitations of everyday life to a level where the senses are so heightened that inanimate objects suddenly seem to have a life force of their own, where sounds take on a new dimension and colours have a richness never perceived before, and where there seems no limit to one's powers of creativity and achievement. Life becomes a roller coaster, fast and exciting, and there are no bounds to the exuberance and energy felt. But recklessness and confusion eventually take over. Crazy, you say? Well, maybe so, but it happens to many sane and intelligent people.

Just as quickly a person can be plunged into the deepest depression and beyond, to a level unknown to most, emptied of all emotion except anguish, where the brain cannot process incoming information from the senses, where normal bodily functions are impaired, and where there is no sense of a future. Only the black despair of the present and a tormenting guilt over past transgressions are given to endure.

To merely say one's mood is altered is not a sufficient description of the illness. The physical effects, too, are many and exhausting, and the sufferer naturally feels bewildered and frightened, ashamed, not understanding why it is happening, and battling to come to terms with its effects. Family and friends are also unable to understand and so confusion reigns and conflicts arise.

These disorders cannot be cured, but fortunately they are readily treatable today, in that Lithium, antidepressant and anticonvulsant medications will help diminish acute episodes and prevent or curb repeated episodes, while psychotherapy will help the individual recognise the signs of a looming episode and deal with the bewilderment, frustration and other personal and social problems.

Knowledge is the first step. The individual and family members should learn as much as possible about the illness, the warning signs of an impending episode, the medications, and what therapy and support groups are available.

Studies suggest that not all people who suffer depression will have a recurrence, but that a large percentage will have at least one subsequent episode in their lifetime. Some people have many episodes. It has been shown that bipolar illness is definitely a recurrent disorder, often starting in teenage years.

Mood regulates how we think, act and behave, helping us participate in life in an acceptable, well-adjusted manner. If mood is lowered to a negative, pessimistic level, a person may not realise his or her full potential, and if the mood then becomes depressed he or she will withdraw from life. On the other hand, when mood is elevated to great optimism, a person may take too many chances, placing her- or himself in jeopardy, and should the mood then become manic the over-exuberance and sense of self-importance will cause reckless, even dangerous, acts, or the behaviour may become intrusive. The individual may drive dangerously, become irritable, angry, or even violent to some degree.

But it is more than mood and behaviour that are affected. It is definitely a 'whole body' illness. This is confirmed by Dr Jay Amsterdam of the University of Pennsylvania who is quoted by Gloria Hochman in *A Brilliant Madness* as saying the illness 'reflects defects in the hormonal system that regulates body function, in the brain neurotransmitters that send messages from cell to cell, and in daily body rhythms', such as the rhythm of waking and sleeping, and the seasonal rhythms. With regard to the hormonal system, the thyroid gland (which produces the hormone thyroxine) is often found to be malfunctioning, many sufferers have increased levels of the stress-related hormone cortisol, and countless women have complained that their symptoms worsen at particular times during their menstrual cycle.

Depression is more than a mood of anguish, despair and loss, or the inability to experience pleasure. There are many physical side effects such as those described on pages 60–61. Changes in eating patterns also take their toll on the body – some over-eat, particularly sweets and carbohydrates (which is common in bipolar disorder) while others lose their appetite and suffer weight loss. A great deal of weight can be either lost or gained, affecting both physical well-being and self-esteem.

This is an illness that can take a person from high to low and back again, over and over. It is physically exhausting, emotionally demoralising and draining, and mentally depleting, whilst it has a hold. And even when the person recovers, the ordeal is not over. She then has to reach out to the world once more, slowly retrain herself as to what is reality and what is not in relation to moods and thoughts, regain self-esteem and confidence, and interact with family, friends and work colleagues.

How the illness affects people differs greatly. Most manic-depressive sufferers' moods level out between their periods of disordered mood, but some are never free of lingering symptoms, while others only have one or two episodes in a lifetime. Of course, there are many others who never seek treatment, perhaps not realising it is possible, or considering it a sign of weakness to seek professional help. So they continue to suffer alone, with no end in sight, until the episode lifts of its own accord.

Some severely depressed people suffer paranoid symptoms, hallucinations, and delusions. They may be so overpowered by a sense of guilt or evil that they firmly believe everybody is out to harm them. Typically, delusions and hallucinations tend to focus on such things as disease, punishment and death, doom and destruction. Sufferers may be convinced that some life-threatening disease is racking their body or that they must suffer some horrible torture and punishment to atone for their wickedness. They may believe that they are hearing the voice of God condemning them for their evil.

Because episodes of severe depression can last for several months or longer, self-esteem can be so severely eroded, and guilt feelings so excessive, that suicide is often contemplated, even attempted. At this point it is good for us to remember that the suicidal person is no longer thinking rationally.

Depression can strike anyone, at any time, at any age. But if it is recognised early and treatment obtained, the acute episodes can be eased, and further episodes can be prevented or controlled. While some people are treatment-resistant (see pages 61–62) and their depression lingers on for a longer period, *all* depressions eventually run their course.

In the following, very touching excerpts from the diary of a 'very young' 66-year-old journalist and grandmother, you will see how Helen's pain and anguish could have been eased had the correct diagnoses of manic-depressive illness been made earlier, and how Lithium was responsible for restoring balance to her life.

December – Family and friends were preaching 'count your blessings, you have a lot to be thankful for'. So I would go for a walk in the late afternoons, wandering around the neighbourhood streets unseeingly, and thinking to myself, 'I have a good husband, three wonderful adult children and four beautiful grandchildren. Yes, I have a lot to be thankful for.' Somehow it made no difference, I just felt the same, which was blackly depressed. How did my breakdown start? I realise one thing with clarity, had I known what was ahead of me for the next year, the living hell I would experience, I would have gone immediately for help!

… I started to wonder if I had been doing too much. Was on the committee of two writers' groups, helped edit a magazine, wrote Neighbourhood Watch newsletter, involved in local Council affairs, and helped at a Day Care Centre for the elderly. I also helped a young lass of whom I was very fond, who had been diagnosed as schizophrenic. I listened to her and started to feel that my symptoms were identical! How did I survive Christmas? No joy …

January – Feelings of inadequacy were stronger than ever. Can't knit like grandchildren's other grandma, can't sew like sister-in-law, can't cook like husband's relations … and should have said *used* to be a writer, as there was absolutely nothing there. I had frightening nightmares, would always dream that 'they' were coming to get me and if they got to the bed, that was the end of me. I started to wake each day with sick feeling of worry.

February – I went to my local doctor and suggested I needed a psychologist to sort myself out, but he referred me to a psychiatrist … who took all my history, and prescribed antidepressant tranquillisers to be taken nightly. I have always been anti-drug and felt reluctant to take them, but I *had* to get better.

March – I would hardly leave the house. I used to look out the window and think 'life is different out there, all those people are normal, not like me'. I used to pray each morning as I wakened, 'Please dear Lord, make me better', but felt He was not hearing me. My husband became my watch-dog, and was hardly absent from home the whole time of my illness.

April – Our younger son's wedding. I bought an expensive outfit, on impulse with my daughter's help. I could not have gone and chosen it by myself. I paid three times as much for it than anything else I have ever bought. Somehow, it didn't worry me. I hardly remember the air flight … and don't know how I got through the wedding. The house … seemed to be packed with people coming and going the whole time we were there and I couldn't keep up with it… By midnight I felt I could stand little more. I looked at my son, the groom, and felt an incredible pain of sadness.

May – I was gradually, no dramatically, getting worse. When we went shopping, I felt everyone was staring at me … Harder and harder to choose food. I would stand in the supermarket in a trance. My husband started to take half a Valium before our weekly excursion to calm himself for the ordeal. Tried to make out a weekly shopping list, but all I could think of every week was 'lettuce and tomatoes'. When he started to go shopping alone, I felt another little slice of my independence was stolen from me.

June – Winter arrived, I felt worse. Came to hate visitors, just couldn't handle them. Tension was terrible. Could hardly communicate even with my young grandchildren. Had always been on very happy wavelength with children, and written stories for them. Every household task seemed major. Meals were basic, I don't know how I managed. I started to cut down on laundry, even rationed how many hankies and tea towels we would use per week. If clothes didn't dry, a major disaster.

July – Tried to sleep some afternoons, as I was having less sleep every night. As I wakened, ungodly feeling of terror and panic enveloped me. Felt that no one out of an asylum could ever experience this. Would jump out of bed and rush to my husband, cling onto him, or run down back of the garden, or pick up a broom and frantically sweep until the panic was gone. Every time I vacuumed, I would mentally assert that this would probably be the last time I would be doing it … Gave husband instructions re washing machine, iron, fridge and defrosting, and where the bed linen lived. Coerced him into having authority to sign and draw on my bank accounts, also told him that if anything happened to me, I wanted a private funeral, no friends, no flowers. Had husband take me to buy new slippers, bras, undies, hair-brush in case I had to go away – to where?

August – More and more difficult to choose what to wear each morning. Each night I would mentally program clothes for next day, but unsuccessfully. Down to two winter outfits. Would pace back and forwards from bedroom to kitchen each morning before dressing trying to decide 'what to wear'. I decided not to overdose on sleeping tablets, as a nurse I knew said the ones I was prescribed would make a person sick, but would not kill. One night my husband was out, I deliberated for an hour with a bottle of drain cleaner in my hand. Put a few crystals on my fingers and into my mouth. It burnt. I realised then, how hellishly it would burn internally. I felt a coward. Could no longer even read the newspaper. Felt sadder and sadder for my husband and family, felt they would be better without me. My hair had lost its lustre, was falling out, and my skin was terrible. I had lost weight, my face was worry-drawn, and nails had developed nasty, fungal ridges.

September – Several times, set clock for 4 a.m., had showered, washed my hair, put on fresh nightgown, toilet bag was packed. Did I think I was going to die or end up in hospital?

October – Finally, my daughter and son went to see my psychiatrist, asking could they get a second opinion. He agreed. My daughter made an appointment for me with a professor of psychiatry. After speaking with me, he called my husband in and told him I was manic-depressive, something of which we had never heard. He prescribed therapeutic Lithium for me, a naturally occurring metallic substance found in sea rocks and mineral springs and not addictive. Within days of using it, the world looked different. I started to think clearly and calmly. Could choose clothes again, everything in the wardrobe felt new, I had forgotten half of what I had. My grandchildren looked like angels, I felt no panic when they came, and I realised how mighty my husband had been and felt my darling daughter had helped save my life.

November and December – Still improving. Starting to bake cakes again … everything looks beautiful and rosy to me. Have trees always been so green and flowers so colourful? Won't need husband to come shopping with me much longer. Can drive the car and manage everything myself. Starting to see my worthwhile qualities again, fostering my self-esteem. I will look into a mirror and think 'I love you'. Looking back and reading my diary, I can see the humour and also the black tragedy which enmeshed my life all those months. Did I really experience it all? It's early December, making Christmas puddings. Will have the family home for Christmas dinner. I CAN COPE.

Helen had one further episode, approximately one year after the conclusion of those diary entries, but following electroconvulsive therapy (ECT) treatment and some antidepressant medication, is now enjoying better health, writing, and again involved in community matters.

One point that should be made here is that, even with this illness, there are positive elements. Whilst it is known that severe depression and mania can disable a person completely or cause utter chaos, in the milder stages of depression and hypomania a person can actually achieve enormous creative output and productivity. The lives of people such as Winston Churchill and Vincent van Gogh are a great testament to this fact.

There are many degrees of depression, both in depression resulting from external causes and in manic-depressive illness, but to be considered an illness, certain symptoms must be present and must have persisted for at least several weeks.

Symptoms of depression

Although the symptoms can vary from person to person, the following are generally those of a clinical depression:

- depressed or irritable mood most of the day
- poor appetite and weight loss, or the opposite, increased appetite and weight gain
- sleep disturbance: sleeping too little, or sleeping too much in an irregular pattern
- loss of energy: excessive fatigue or tiredness
- change in activity level, either increased or decreased
- loss of interest or pleasure in usual activities
- decreased sexual drive
- diminished ability to think or concentrate

- feelings of worthlessness or excessive guilt that may reach grossly unreasonable or delusional proportions
- recurrent thoughts of death or self-harm, wishing to be dead or contemplating or attempting suicide

If at least five of these symptoms have been present almost every day for a two-week period, one of them being either depressed mood or loss of interest or pleasure, then medical help should be sought immediately.

Symptoms of mania and hypomania

In contrast to depression, the symptoms of mania and hypomania are as follows:
- persistently 'high' (euphoric) and/or irritable mood states
- decreased need for sleep
- appetite disturbance
- increased activity, sociability and sexual drive
- pressured speech
- racing thoughts
- loss of self-control and judgment

Subtypes of manic-depressive illness

There are several subtypes of manic-depressive illness that should be mentioned.

Mixed states

A person is said to be in a mixed state when significant symptoms of both mania and depression are present at the same time. Treatment for these people is often more difficult than for those who have their manic and depressive episodes well apart.

An example of this state could be when a person displays the restlessness and heightened libido that accompany a manic episode, while at the same time experiencing an undercurrent of gloomy mood and discontent.

Rapid cycling

Between five and twenty per cent of bipolar sufferers, mostly women, are rapid cyclers. These people are so categorised because they experience frequent recurrences of depression and mania on a regular and continuing basis. A rapid cycler's mood swings dramatically in cycles which could be daily, weekly or monthly. However, the shorter mood swings typically occur in the context of an illness that has included longer episodes as well. Those who experience regular episodes of depression, mania or hypomania, with the episodes occurring more than four times in one year, fall into the category of rapid cycling.

The National Depressive and Manic-Depressive Association (Chicago), in its brochure *In Bipolar Illness: Rapid Cycling & Its Treatment,* points out that studies have shown that it occurs more frequently in people with bipolar disorders who have evidence or a history of hypothyroidism, and in those who have relatives suffering from affective disorders. There is also a possible genetic or other physiological link between rapid cycling and drug or alcohol abuse, with some studies indicating that substance abuse is more common in families of those with rapid cycling illness than in families of bipolar patients without rapid cycling. In some people, rapid cycling is evident from the beginning of their illness, while in others the onset is gradual.

Treatment for these people can be difficult due to the sudden, unpredictable mood changes, and the fact that the response rate to Lithium in these sufferers is only twenty to forty per cent, compared to approximately seventy per cent in other sufferers. But anticonvulsant medication has more recently proved very beneficial.

Rhonda experienced the usual symptoms of the illness in her depressive and manic states, with fortnightly cycles. She was regularly high for two weeks, then low for two weeks. But even knowing that her depression would lift at the end of the fortnight did not help her when the depression was deep. She said, 'You can't make yourself feel better, can't smile or pretend to be happy, you feel weighed down with problems, feel as though you've always been this way and always will – even though you know it will only last for two weeks.'

And then, two weeks later: 'Everything is wonderful, I want to party and be with people all the time. I feel that I can change things with the sheer force of my personality.'

Rhonda goes on to tell us of her experiences, starting when she first suspected that something was wrong.

I think every individual's experience, treatment and management has to be looked at in conjunction with the probable cause. In my own case, I would say I had a less powerful genetic predisposition to bipolar disorder, and that my illness was induced by stress and environmental factors, and possibly a hormonal cause as the cycles coincided with my menstrual cycle. I have been told that there is a connection between hormonal factors and rapid cyclers.

I was on my way back to Australia after two and a half years travelling overseas. Six months before my return I seemed to be suffering from pre-menstrual syndrome. Just before my return I had a much more serious depression lasting for two weeks, followed immediately by two weeks of being 'high'. The onset coincided with the stress of returning home and settling back into ordinary life with its responsibilities ...

Stage 1 – Before diagnosis

I had continuous cycles of two weeks down followed by two weeks up. There was no transition period. I would go to sleep at the end of a down period and wake up the next morning in a high state. This went on for six months before I was diagnosed. I did not notice the highs so much. My family and friends, who hadn't seen me for years, thought I'd changed and that I was now more animated, confident, up-front and talkative ... I noticed the depressions more, and kept a record of when they occurred, noticing that it was always the week before and the week when I menstruated. I assumed it was severe PMS that was disrupting my life, but no treatments tried for PMS had any effect ...

During the period before diagnosis, I realised that neither of the two states was the 'real' me but, as the months went by, the real me was becoming but a dim memory, and that was scary. As time went on, I couldn't keep denying that the high and low periods weren't the real me because that was all I had, and I had to be one or the other to survive. I felt I had a split personality ...

Once I realised that I was depressed for two weeks out of four, I tried to live my life in the two weeks I had available as a functioning, though high, person. It was exhausting, with little sleep, a lot of socialising, and many ideas and projects on the go. I would apply for jobs I couldn't have reasonably expected to be able to do, but would write confident letters and sometimes be interviewed, although the interviews weren't successful because of the high state I was in ...

I began to notice that the depressions were stopping me from working and getting on with my new life. This deepened my depression. My family was losing patience with me too. They thought I was rude, inconsiderate and overbearing when I was 'up', and expected me to just 'snap out of' my depressions. My social life suffered because old friends didn't really like the new 'up' me. I'd hide away during the low periods, waiting for the mood to pass as it always did, but at times when I was caught up in a depression it really seemed impossible that it would end …

I became tired of waiting to 'settle down', and … after six months, I reached a crisis point and was finally diagnosed.

Stage 2 – Initial treatment
For the next six months, with medication, the cycles continued, but gradually I began to have a respite with two normal-mood days as a transition between cycles …

I had been led to believe that once I was taking Lithium, my mood would be stabilised, and so I was becoming impatient. I was taking a very high dosage, along with Tegretol, a drug which is often successful with rapid cyclers. I experienced some of the usual side effects of these drugs, but the most debilitating side effect was a feeling of 'fogginess' of the mind. It was a struggle to achieve any mental clarity, let alone try to concentrate or remember things.

Towards the end of the first six months of treatment I consulted a naturopath/counsellor to deal with this fogginess. After a few weeks of using homeopathic medicines which are used in cyclic illnesses, the fogginess disappeared, and instead of having up and down cycles, I had 'flat' periods (slightly depressed) interspersed with two days of normal mood …

Stage 3 – Stability
The next six months was a period of stability with these 'flat' periods for two weeks, then two days of normal mood. I continued taking the medication in high doses, together with homeopathic medicine to combat the accompanying low levels of energy. I was feeling flat and lethargic most of the time and did not feel connected to what was going on around me. However, I did manage to work, and although it was manual, mindless work, it showed that I was at least able to lead a 'normal' life. Although, to me, it was more like existing, not living.

I had to be very patient, to see what progress was made over time. My naturopath suggested I keep a diary and note down such things as what I was doing and thinking, my diet, exercise and sleeping habits. He also asked me to rate my mood and energy each day on a scale of 1 to 5. By referring to this I could see that things were slowly improving in my mood and memory, but the tiredness still remained. One of the most difficult things about feeling 'not myself' for so long was that I couldn't rely on my perceptions to gauge my progress. My 'indicators', apart from my thoughts and my diary, were other people's perceptions, the levels of my sociability, confidence, anxiety and panic, and the more positive feelings which I had for the future.

At the end of this stage, when asked to rate my well-being from 0 (lowest) to 10 (before illness), I rated myself as 8. I was stable and functioning. When my naturopath asked, 'Who got you from 0 to 8?' I realised that, apart from him, my psychiatrist, family and friends, I had done a lot to help myself get to this stage.

Stage 4 – Improvement

I felt as though I had reached the end of a particular stage. My mood was stable, though still flat, I was functioning in the world, and although I was prone to anxiety and found it difficult to control my emotions when stressed, I was at about eighty per cent of my old self …

Meanwhile, I had lost a lot of confidence, self-esteem, time, friends and also hope and optimism for the future … I felt in a state of limbo …

My naturopath suggested that I achieve what I'm capable of now, and then move on to the next stage without thinking of my end position …

Once stable, I now had to look at my core, that is to explore my feelings and problems to discover what had caused the illness. In doing this it was an opportunity to know myself and grow. I had to recognise my tolerance to different stressors, accept my limitations, and look after myself by avoiding, as far as possible, stressful people and situations. I had to give myself permission to live within these limitations and not to compare myself and my life to what it had previously been. With an idea of my present capabilities and revised goals, over the following year I found a job which suited me and which I could handle and, along with improvements in my living situation and social life, I felt I had achieved my aims, felt comfortable with my new self, and so regained my self-esteem and feelings of well-being.

Stage 5 – Recovery

My psychiatrist, naturopath/counsellor and I all believe that I am now recovered and, because the set of circumstances which triggered the illness initially was a one-off situation, it seems unlikely that the illness will recur as long as I maintain my current lifestyle and remain aware that I am prone to suffering from stress.

Cyclothymia

Some people experience mood swings that are more extreme than normal but not extreme enough to be considered manic-depressive illness. They are diagnosed as suffering from cyclothymia. These swings can and do interfere with everyday life and relationships as the person alternates from feeling helpless and inadequate to being overactive and over-confident, but the episodes are short and irregular.

Charting the mood and course of the illness

Many psychiatrists ask their patients to keep a graph of their moods on a daily basis. This is to enable the psychiatrist to follow the course the illness is taking. Often, if your visits are fortnightly or monthly, you may well forget to acquaint him or her of something important that has happened, but if you have kept a chart with accompanying brief notes, it acts as a prompt to your psychiatrist to ask pertinent questions should there be any sharp fluctuations recorded that may necessitate a change in medication. It also enables you both to look back from time to time and make an accurate appraisal of your progress.

Below is a sample of the manner in which I kept my graph. It starts at the bottom with 00 which represents the deepest suicidal despair of major depression, and works its way up through the various stages of depression and feeling 'blue' to 100, which is a normal day. Anything over 100 represents an elevated mood, hypomania, and eventually mania.

Charting the mood

September

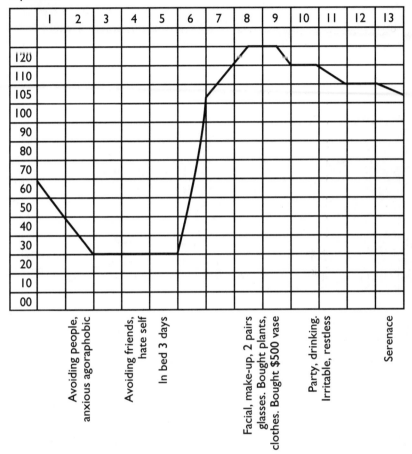

The graph provides a description of what will be happening to the person with each different level of mood, starting with black depression at 00, working up to normal mood at 100, and then continuing on upwards into mania.

Scale of mood		Symptoms
Severe mania psychosis	140	Grandiose delusions, hallucinations Thoughts chaotic, speech jumbled
Mania	120	Delusions, highly responsive and receptive, feel 'at one' with world and universe, euphoric, all senses heightened, pressured speech, flights of ideas
	110	Excessive spending, gross indiscretions, poor concentration and focus, no sleep needed
Hypomania	105	Boundless energy, infectious exuberance, racing thoughts and actions, little sleep
	102	Over-excited, creative, don't tire, 'high' Feel excited, exuberant, loads of energy Feel happy, confident, 'great to be alive'
Healthy mood	**100**	**Normal mood = Average day**
	90	Feel ordinary most of the time
	80	A little under par, less energy and interest
	70	'Down in the dumps', low energy, may cry occasionally
Depressed	60	Depressed from time to time, not very interested in life or people, low on energy, cry a lot
'Grey' clinical depression	50	Longer episode of depression, lose confidence and self-respect, will shut yourself away from everyone, go to bed, world looks grey and bleak, appetite and sleeping patterns changed, aches, pains, constipation
	40	World looks grey for longer periods, no energy, dwell on past
	30	Future looks bleak
'Black' clinical depression	20	Devoid of feeling except hopelessness, helplessness, self-loathing, guilt

	10 Complete loss of concentration, memory, general functioning.
	00 There seems to be no future, world looks black, thoughts of suicide.
Psychotic depression	Delusions, out of touch with reality, hallucinations

In trying to visualise these mood fluctuations, it may help if you liken the moods to an elevator shaft, where ground floor equates to normal mood and each floor above or below equates to a steady change in mood, either up or down.

In depression, the elevator descends below ground level, through each floor, or mood change, until it finally reaches the lowest level which is severe psychotic depression.

Above ground level, the elevator rides upwards, going higher and higher through each level or mood change, until it reaches the top floor which represents severe mania psychosis.

My own graphs, along with the notes and journal kept throughout my illness, have all helped me gain a better understanding of the illness, greater self-awareness and, ultimately, greater self-acceptance.

7 Causes of manic-depressive illness

Enormous progress has been made in the study of the major affective disorders during the past decade, and yet there still seems to be no simple clear-cut answer to the questions: what causes manic-depressive illness, and who is most likely to develop it?

There seems to be little doubt, however, among mental health experts that certain forms of depression and manic-depressive illness are biochemical illnesses. They know that manic-depressive illness runs in families, that there is a genetic factor, and that there may be some relationship between genetics and environment that influences the development and course of the illness. It is considered to be a genetically determined disorder which can be, but is not always, induced by stress or other environmental factors. However, the disorder often occurs spontaneously, not precipitated by any external cause.

The question of nature or nurture seems to be the subject of much debate – that is, whether the disorder occurs as a result of inheriting a faulty gene, or of growing up in a family where the previous generation had sufferers, or a combination of both.

Many studies have been done, including incidence of the disorder in identical twins compared with non-identical twins. These studies offer the most compelling evidence that genetics and mood disorders go together. Because identical twins have exactly the same genes, they would be expected to inherit the same predisposition to an illness, whereas non-identical twins are no more the same genetically than are any brothers and sisters. Studies have shown that in identical twins there is a far greater incidence of both twins developing the illness than in non-identical twins, whether they are reared by their natural parents or by adoptive parents who have no family history of the disorder.

The task of searching for the faulty gene, or genes, has been going on for many years, and it has recently been discovered that there is at least one, but probably more than one, abnormal gene responsible for causing manic-depressive illness. Many researchers believe the X chromosome is involved, while chromosome 11 could be another.

Gloria Hochman in *A Brilliant Madness* mentions a 1969 research project where it was found, in two families, that everyone who was colour-blind also had manic-depressive illness. It was concluded that the gene for colour blindness, which is located at the bottom of the X chromosome, must be very close to a gene for manic-depression. Another study of five large families in Jerusalem also found that in forty-seven people there was that same link between colour blindness (and anaemia), and manic-depressive illness on the X chromosome. Dr Neil Risch of the Yale University School of Medicine, one of the investigators, said that a substantial number of the cases of manic-depressive illness are probably linked to a defect on the X chromosome.

There are, however, other factors to consider. Some people develop the disorder where there is no related family history. Dr David Grounds and June Armstrong suggest in *Ecstasy & Agony* that 'spontaneous mutation of a gene may be one cause for this, or alternatively a disease, which itself is not genetically determined, may develop in the brain and cause *mood disorder*' ('mood disorder' is an authors' correction made since the publication of *Ecstasy & Agony*).

Dr Janice Egeland, a medical sociologist at the University of Miami School of Medicine, following a study of three generations of a number of Amish families, announced in 1987 that there was an identifiable defect near the top of chromosome 11, although more extensive research since that time has failed to conclusively prove this. There are many researchers continuing this important work in the hope of identifying other abnormal gene locations or at least confirming the findings to date relating to chromosome 11 or the X chromosome.

Many people inherit a faulty gene but do not develop the illness, so there are obviously other factors involved. It has been suggested that personality may play a part – for instance, a person who is predisposed to developing this illness for other reasons and also has a tendency to be moody, with periods of sluggishness and unhappiness alternating with periods of high animation, is more at risk of developing bipolar disorder. The creative personality has also been shown to be at risk, such as in writers, poets, artists, actors and musicians.

It has also been suggested that the increased use of alcohol and illicit drugs may interact in some way with a genetic vulnerability.

Stressful events and loss, or events that equate with loss, can precipitate an attack. The stressors could be anything from the break-up of a relationship, or illness, to driving oneself too hard at work, or entering a new relationship.

Research by Dr Robert Post, chief of the biological psychiatry branch of the National Institute of Mental Health, USA, suggests that psychological and social stressors not only affect neurotransmitters in the brain and the endocrine system, but also alter the way genes are expressed and cause a long-lasting change that results in vulnerability to manic or depressive episodes.

There would also appear to be a definite hormonal component of manic-depressive illness, with childbirth and the time around menopause also having been shown to be triggers for episodes of the illness.

It has also been suggested by many that the illness is perhaps linked with a disturbance of the body's biological clocks which control the timing of the various bodily rhythms or cycles, in relation to each other and in relation to conditions in the environment such as the day/night cycle. This could explain why so many depressed sufferers report that their symptoms are worse in the morning, while their energy levels increase during the afternoon, and it would certainly account for the changes in sleeping patterns. Changes in seasons can also precipitate episodes in some people, although many of these people are said to be suffering seasonal affective disorder (SAD), and may not necessarily be considered to be suffering from manic-depressive illness.

The chemical factor

Mood, actions, thought, memory, sensations, and so on are controlled in the brain by electrochemical interactions. Messages are passed from our external senses to the relevant part of the brain and then on to our consciousness, or awareness. The limbic system of the brain, which is concerned with mood, then receives a message and we feel pleasure or pain, etc. The message then travels down the nerve cell as an electric current, to be passed on to the next cell.

The brain consists of many millions of these nerve cells, each conducting tiny electric charges to others. Between cells are microscopic gaps called synapses. The electric current cannot jump the synapse, but instead causes a change in the chemicals within the synapse; this change then causes a current to start in the head of the next cell. These chemicals are called neurotransmitters because they transmit the electrical charge from one cell to the next. Many neurotransmitters have been discovered, so it is difficult to know which causes what effect, but the ones mainly concerned with mood are noradrenaline, serotonin and dopamine.

Changes occur in the amounts of these neurotransmitters during mania and depression, causing mood to be altered. The use of various drugs, however, has been shown to change the level of neurotransmitters, and to control the mood disorder.

The creative factor

Before going any further, I would like to mention the term 'nervous breakdown' – a term loosely used by lay people to cover the broad spectrum of disorders that arise in the body when a person is considered to be 'out of control', no longer able to cope. It is not a medical definition as such, but does cover anxiety and depression. It does not include the mental illnesses manic-depression and schizophrenia.

People from all walks of life suffer breakdowns and mental illness, but the creative temperament of artistic people seems to destine them to a fairly high proportion of such illnesses. Creative people are often more attuned to the way they think and feel and the way others think and feel, with the result that they tend to be more introspective and more easily led into depression by self-analysis. Spike Milligan, who openly talked of his illness, once said, 'You get the pain much worse than anyone else, but you see a sunrise much more beautiful than anybody else.' Such people, by their very nature, tend to be sensitive, and are more likely to carry emotional reactions and human interactions to a much deeper level. They are also more vulnerable to emotional storms and, it seems, to manic-depressive illness, depression and 'nervous breakdowns'.

Many highly creative, gifted and famous people throughout the centuries have suffered from manic-depressive illness, yet managed somehow to continue with their important work. They include King Saul of the Bible, King George III, George Frederick Handel, Abraham

Lincoln, Theodore Roosevelt, Winston Churchill, Ernest Hemingway, Virginia Woolf, Vivien Leigh, Spike Milligan, Connie Francis and Tony Hancock. More recently, Patty Duke Austin has written of her experiences and how, with Lithium, she has gained control of her life. Her book *My Brilliant Madness* provides a wealth of hope and encouragement for others affected by this illness.

Tim Finn told Lina Safro, doctor-turned-documentary film-maker in 'The Darkness Within' by Janet Hawley, (*Good Weekend*, 29 April 1995) that he does his best work when coming out of depression, and knows of many singers, songwriters, painters and other artists who sense, consciously or subconsciously, that this dark side helps their creative process. I relate to this interesting statement, although I find that the work done when coming out of a depressive state, whilst being full of great insight, is also very melancholy.

Rilke, the German poet, refused psychoanalysis from Freud with his legendary quote: 'If you exorcise my demons, my angels might leave as well.'

As Dr Safro says in 'The Darkness Within', 'Depression can shape people's lives, colour their work, but it can also destroy them. It is a proven lethal illness. And yet, depression remains the hidden epidemic of Western society ...'

8 The course of my illness

The illness that began with my first anxiety attack in the spring of 1987 was to continue in its various phases for eight years. I had no idea, at the end of 1988, that I was not even halfway along the road that manic-depressive illness was going to take me.

1989

By February 1989 I was about three stone (nineteen kilograms) overweight, and being all of five feet (154 centimetres) tall, I could not afford to carry so much excess weight. I decided to stop the antidepressant Sinequan and see if my weight dropped back. I thought my mood to be about seventy per cent normal at that stage and felt that I could cope without medication. To be depressed was bad enough, but to be fat and depressed was more than I could bear. Dr W. pointed out matter-of-factly that the depression itself, not just the Sinequan, might be causing me to eat so much, and that this was common.

I have proved, on both that and a future occasion, that Sinequan was responsible for a good deal of weight gain. However, it was certainly a pity I stopped taking it at that particular time, because it was the only antidepressant throughout the years of my deepest depressions that caused a marked improvement in my condition. But I felt strongly that I had to take whatever measures I could to lose some of the weight that was causing my intense self-loathing. I continued on with Lithium and Oroxine, but only a few weeks had passed when each day saw me slipping into a deeper, darker depression.

I had now reached the next stage of depression where every moment spent in the company of others was exhausting and left me feeling very anxious. So I turned to my own company more and more, often becoming resentful when someone intruded on my thoughts, my privacy. I did not want pity, or even sympathy for that matter. What I really did need was genuine acceptance and understanding.

Dr W. discussed with me the possibility of other antidepressants that did not have the unwanted side effect of weight gain. And so began a merry-go-round of different medications. Although the depression was severe, there was the usual ebb and flow as various antidepressants provided some relief from time to time. But there was none that worked as well as the Sinequan had.

Some months later, the depression seemed to have lifted markedly. In fact, I was feeling remarkably good. What I did not realise was that I was now experiencing hypomanic episodes along with the symptoms of depression, which accounted for much of my happier, more confident disposition. In fact, this condition, known as a 'mixed state', had been going on for some time. I just assumed that these were 'normal' periods because I felt so good, and would tell Dr W. that I was feeling close to normal with just a low-grade depression.

At that time I had never heard of the word manic, so many events in my life that I considered to be normal I obviously did not mention to my doctor. By the time it was discovered that I was having these episodes, I was re-classified as manic-depressive instead of as suffering from unipolar depression. Some of the highs at that stage may have been induced by withdrawing from antidepressant medication, but certainly not all of them were.

In depression, the libido is one of the first things to scuttle out the door. But when a person is 'high', the libido comes banging on the door again, demanding attention, and often running amuck. And that's what happened to me at this time. No matter what the mirror told me, I thought I had the appeal of Elle Macpherson.

At this end of the bipolar scale as the mood swings upwards, the hypomanic person feels wonderful and very confident. Hypomania is the first stage, or a more controlled state, of mania. A person experiencing hypomania is usually said to be high, feeling excited, more creative, intelligent and sexual than ever before, believing they have reached the height of all their powers. Little or no sleep is needed, and the person is often headstrong, impatient and manipulative, with an uncanny ability to exert control over other people. This state produces boundless energy and enthusiasm, and self-confidence is so great that there is a sense of enormous power and purpose. The mood becomes euphoric.

Activity level increases, and there is a restlessness, an urge to keep moving. With no more need for sleep, a person can be up all night working, or with even two to four hours' sleep wake energetic and eager to pursue the day's activities. This pattern can continue for many days. Sleeping patterns are a good indicator of whether the mood is going up or down, and it is important to be watchful in this regard. Abundant energy around the clock with the inability to sleep are sure signs that a manic phase has been entered.

As the mood elevates, the person develops an infectious sense of humour. The mind is flooded with idea after idea that catches the fancy, and jokes and puns can come pouring out one after the other. At times they may be totally inappropriate, causing some embarrassment when the mood returns to normal.

There is often a great urge to create and achieve – it could be composing music, writing a book, re-decorating the house or working on some new invention – and the person is literally driven by an uncontrollable force to work mentally and physically at a constant and frenzied pace. A small high can produce excellent work, but often, in the higher manic state, the work will reflect the frenzied state of mind. Once the manic episode has subsided, the person can suffer an awful internal humiliation when faced with reality, with the fact of natural talents and limitations, as well as the realisation that he or she not only had grandiose ideas, but must now again deal with the fact of mental illness.

During a manic phase there is also a great need to make human contact – with anyone and everyone. The person becomes overly sociable, wanting to touch everyone, to hug and kiss, and even to make such contact with strangers on the street. Quite often people are attracted to, or at least intrigued by, this effervescence.

Many people in this state find themselves impetuously taking up excessive letter-writing or spending hours and hours on the telephone, sometimes calling interstate or overseas, often at all hours of the night, without any thought of time or cost.

Rhonda tells us how being high caused her dismissal from her new job:

> I'd had the interview when I was in a low cycle, but when I started the job the following week I was in a high …

Because of the previous sleepless night I made numerous trips to the coffee machine. I became aggressive, telling everyone how disgraceful it was to be using foam cups, and I pinned up a note telling people to bring their own coffee mugs. At the same time I voted myself in for the job of organising the recycling of paper ...

I chatted loudly and at length all day, and at the end of the day walked down to the elevator, still talking. I noticed that people were staring at me ...

The next morning I was warned by my boss to quieten down and let the others get on with their work ...

Realising I had been talking too much, the following day I brought my Walkman in with me, but I ended up doing a bit of singing and dancing ... So, at the end of my second day I was given a final warning – settle down tomorrow or lose my job.

After all the highs and lows of the previous six months I really needed to keep this job, to get my life going again, and I was determined that I would not be sacked. So, on my third day I brought classical music with me ... But somehow it was all beyond my control. There was a Groucho Marx mask lying around ... I put it on, grabbed a feather duster, and began waving it through the window to the people on the construction site next door. Then I stuck funny notes in big letters onto the windows for the builders to laugh at ...

By lunchtime I had been fired, and I could almost hear the whole office sigh with relief as I walked out the door.

My exuberance, too, was at times quite over the top. I enjoyed life to the hilt in every way, drinking too much, still overweight, still feeling like Elle. This feeling was brought about by another phase of the illness which has a great potential for distaster. The heightening of libido, combined with the recklessness that accompanies manic episodes, can lead to unexpected sexual behaviour. 'Falling in love' and pursuing an affair or affairs is common, without discrimination. This need for promiscuity is fuelled by an uncontrollable driving force, so it is important that these episodes be recognised and help sought immediately.

I was still experiencing some highs, although I was more often in a 'mixed state' with the underlying discontent and agitation of depression. At this stage I did not understand the details of the hypomanic state, and did not discuss certain aspects of my illness with my doctor.

There can be a heightening of all the senses in this state, and a feeling of being at one with the universe. I enjoyed some of these sensations enormously, believing that because I was so happy and the world so beautiful, I must have at last been cured. Colours were so vibrant and rich that I saw them as if for the first time, wondering that I had never noticed this richness before. Surfaces were more textural to the touch, inanimate objects took on a life force I was completely in tune with, and suddenly I was hearing all sounds in what could only be described as stereo-sensurround. It was like being re-born, discovering the world for the first time.

I remember one evening, leaning over a balcony at a friend's home, looking at the side wall of very ordinary double-storey flats next door. On this particular evening they exuded a very appealing mystery and charm. The building seemed to be beckoning me over to participate in some kind of interchange of thoughts and feelings. It had its own very real life force and we belonged together in our own world.

So, along with my memories of depression to give my future life more depth, I would now also carry memories of a very special moment in time when a block of flats was no longer just a block of flats.

All of my senses became heightened during these episodes, and a journal entry shows what I mean:

> The leaves on the peppercorn are light and feathery, tickled by the breeze. They're playing joyfully, teasing the chimney. The chimney has an aura around it, and it's reaching out to touch the leaves. I can feel the life, the energy in the chimney, in everything out there, and I'm part of it.

There's an energy stirring deep inside me, surging to the surface. Joe is hammering away next door again, but today it doesn't bother me. It's a vibrant ringing that I hear as he pushes the nail into its bed. Sounds are so clear today – I can hear in three-D.

Thinking that I was almost back to normal, I decided to look for a job closer to home because of the daily drive over the Westgate Bridge. I was getting up later and later as the months went by, finding it difficult to get to work by eight. So I applied for a job only five minutes from home, was successful, and started working there in May 1989, confident that I was well on the road to complete recovery.

Early in June 1989 I was hospitalised for further surgery on my leg. There was a large crater just above the knee where the melanoma had been removed, and the plastic surgeon had to reconstruct the area. The complete bed rest for two weeks had a very calming effect and I left the hospital feeling like a new person. When I resumed work, George drove me there and back while I was still on crutches. My panic attacks eased off, and this gave me further time to recuperate mentally and physically.

But the anxiety and panic attacks soon hit with renewed vigour and the new antidepressants seemed to no longer work. I started to descend into an even deeper depression. Many have tried to describe a deep clinical depression as vast emptiness, anguish, agony and despair, but no words adequately portray the depth of the anguish, of the despair, or the immeasurable emptiness, isolation and actual pain, both mental and physical.

Needless to say a great sense of loss accompanies such severe depression. The sufferer mourns the loss of loved ones, the world around them, and the annihilation of self, having become as barren as the vast desert sands mentally, emotionally, physically and spiritually. Every hidden corner of his being has been filled with torment of the worst possible kind. It defies description.

The description given by William James in *The Varieties of Religious Experience* is as good as any I have read: 'It is a positive and active anguish, a sort of psychical neuralgia wholly unknown to normal life.' But James wrote this after giving up the search for an adequate description, implying its near-impossibility.

It is common for the depressed person to see the depression as an invasion by an intruder, an enemy, and even to have an accompanying visual image and a name for it. Winston Churchill, for example, called his depression the 'Black Dog', while William Styron, author of *Sophie's Choice* and *Darkness Visible*, referred to his as 'The Beast'. Tim Finn called his the 'Dirty Creature'. Tim had a nervous breakdown around age thirty with lots of anxiety attacks. He was very edgy and frightened, and by writing his song 'Dirty Creature' he was able to externalise a lot of that fear. Every time he sang it, it was like a catharsis, a release of his fear.

Nada, twenty-three, sees her depression as 'the enemy' lurking within the depths of her mind, and her very moving account echoes the unspoken words of many depressed people:

> The enemy has returned. I feel him lurk within the depths of my mind. He has come to banish the light, to invade my world with darkness.

Choked up cries are emitted from within as I plead for his vengeance to leave me. My will is weakened. My spirit is fading. My body succumbs to his power.

The light has gone and darkness prevails, the air is heavy with his presence. My soul is inflicted with growing pain as his power surges within me.

He stabs my mind with frightening thoughts and plagues it with confusion. He plays on my fears, twists my emotions and questions the worth of my being.

My body trembles from the battle within. My breaths are hard and heavy. I become as a zombie, a sad broken spirit, controlled by a greater power.

My mind is a magnet to pain and sorrow, a magnifying glass to gloom. My eyes see the clouds but are blind to the sun. They see in shades of grey.

He lies deep within me, sapping my energy, inflicting his pain, ready and waiting to come forth, to shatter my dreams and consume my hopes.

The boundaries of my world are constricted, my growth blocked by anguish. My life is so black, my burden so heavy. The light is so far away.

Robert Burton, who himself suffered from melancholy, the name given to the illness before it acquired the rather inadequate title of depression, wrote in his 1621 *Anatomy of Melancholy:*

They are in great pain and horror of mind, distraction of soul, restless, full of continual fears, cares, torment, anxieties, they can neither drink, eat, nor sleep for them, take no rest, neither at bed nor yet at board …

Virginia Woolf wrote in her diary (*'A Writer's Diary': Extracts From the Diary of Virginia Woolf*, edited by Leonard Woolf, The Hogarth Press, London, 1965):

Never was there such aimlessness, such depression. Can't read, write or think … And my brain is extinct – literally hasn't the power to lift a pen … And I'm empty with a cold slab of a brain …

And then I was in 'one of my states' – how violent, how acute – and walked in Regents Park in black misery and had to summon my cohorts in the old way to see me through, which they have done more or less. A note made to testify to my own ups and downs: many of which go unrecorded though they are less violent I think than they used to be. But how familiar it was – stamping along the road, with gloom and pain constricting my heart: and the desire for death, in the old way, all for two I daresay careless words.

William Styron, in his book *Darkness Visible* (Jonathan Cape), tried to find suitable words to describe his depression:

> I was feeling in my mind a sensation close to, but indescribably different from, actual pain. For myself, the pain is most closely connected to drowning or suffocation – but even these images are off the mark …

> … if the pain were readily describable most of the countless sufferers from this ancient affliction would have been able to confidently depict for their friends and loved ones (even their physicians) some of the actual dimensions of their torment, and perhaps elicit a comprehension that has been generally lacking; such incomprehension has usually been due not to a failure of sympathy but to the basic inability of healthy people to imagine a form of torment so alien to everyday experience.

Dr Anthony Clare, in *Depression And How To Survive It,* tells how Dr John Horder, a former President of the Royal College of Practitioners in England, when interviewed by *Medical News*, compared his experiences of pain associated with both a heart attack and an episode of severe depression:

> If I had to choose again, I would prefer to avoid the pain of depression. It is a surprisingly physical sensation, with a surprising resemblance to coronary pain, because it too is total. But it cannot be relieved quickly. It even threatens life. It is oneself and not part of one's machinery – a form of total paralysis of desire, hope, capacity to decide, to do, to think or to feel – except pain and misery.

A sense of isolation was one of the most distinguishing marks of my depression. The other, and the most distressing, was the internal emptiness and desolation. This was a physical feeling of every internal part of my body, as well as my mind, having been scraped away, leaving a hollow shell, devoid of substance and emotion, but filled with a constant harrowing pain. I had repeated visions of a metal instrument with sharp teeth scraping out my body until there was nothing left.

This sense of emptiness particularly convinced me that I was indeed suffering from an illness, that it was not something I could just pull myself out of. But it took twelve months of this desolation before I was able to completely let go and accept my illness for what it was. Prior to that I had always held a glimmer of hope that it might not have been endogenous depression, that I might suddenly and miraculously just 'lift out of it'.

I now began to understand that I had slipped over the boundary from what we commonly term real 'depression' into the world of mental illness – and there is a vast difference. I knew I could not have expected anyone to understand what I was going through, but did my face need to be distorted, my eyes rolling, or my gait noticeably lurching, for someone to believe that something was wrong inside my head?

I was in the grip of something tenacious. Where would I end up? What would happen to my mind? Each day brought changes that made me less and less of a person, as though some force were manipulating my mind and body, taking control and removing pieces as it saw fit. It was the lack of control that finally got to me. Human beings are created with a mind, a soul, and free-will. If those hallmarks of humanity were taken from me forever, I would cease to be. I fought, and fought hard, using every ounce of strength left, forcing my mind to do the daily tasks now virtually beyond its capability. But without a healthy mind to provide the necessary self-motivating thoughts, without a healthy body to provide the energy needed, how could I expect to win my battle against this insidious and horrifying illness?

My family still needed me, and people at work relied on me to do my job. I also felt an obligation to my friends. Many were no longer keeping in touch, maybe because I'd let them down, or because of my outrageous behaviour when I was high. Or maybe they were unsure of how to handle me.

I could no longer derive even the smallest amount of interest or pleasure from anything in life. The chats and good belly-laughs with my girlfriend over coffee were but a dim memory; I tried to recall the 'feeling' of laughter, but it eluded me completely, as though it were something I had once read about but never actually experienced; my hobbies were things of the past, and my favourite TV shows were of such little interest that I closed my eyes to them and slept instead.

In my darkest days, certain very vivid images constantly loomed large. I could see myself having been dumped unceremoniously into a huge dark abyss, in the bowels of hell – alone except for the demons that kept me chained there. Every evening I would curl up for hours in my favourite place, my couch, with my hands clenched into little balls, wanting to scream for help, to be released from my demons. I hoped for a flood of tears to free me, to release the pain, but the tears were dammed deep inside.

Everyone had good advice for me: 'Think positive', 'Get some fresh air and exercise', 'Have a good cry on someone's shoulder'. All very well, except that my normal thought processes no longer worked, and I needed every ounce of strength just to stay alive, to comprehend the mechanics of life going on around me, let alone exercise or cry. So the advice of well-meaning family and friends could not take hold and bear fruit. What I needed, what all depressed people need, was acceptance, to be allowed to suffer this unsolicited illness with dignity. We need to be told, lovingly, that we will not be deserted, that it will not always be this bad, that it will all come to an end one day.

Inevitably there came the usual slowing down in the rate and content of thoughts which causes great consternation for the sufferer who knows that the brain is slowly but surely grinding to a halt, and is acutely aware of a rate of thinking that cannot keep up with others'.

When I reached this stage, when I could no longer decipher what people were saying, I fell into a state of utter helplessness and hopelessness. Skills I had taken for granted disappeared rapidly, one by one. I could no longer locate keys on the typewriter; I was unable to distinguish one letter from another. Writing was also difficult. I was mentally incapable of stringing letters or words together properly, and unable to push the pen.

The sense of hopelessness is the most ominous of the symptoms. The sufferer knows that he is powerless to change his world, and so despair sets in. The present and past are the only worlds open to him and his mind is allowed to see only the negative aspects, which he magnifies out of all proportion. He feels bad, worthless, and a burden to others. These feelings of worthlessness can ultimately lead to attempts at suicide.

One of the most difficult things for anyone else to understand must surely be the inability to imagine a future. Next week? Next month? Next year? I had no concept of them at all. I no longer had an imagination, or a viewpoint, and was completely unable to reason.

My mind and body had now ground slowly to a halt. Movement and speech became very slow, and it took a supreme effort just to exist. I could no longer make even the smallest decisions. To take a towel out of the linen press was a mammoth task fraught with confusion. Colours meant nothing to me any more. I could not describe or name them. Should it be this one or that one? What was the difference between them anyway?

It was the same dressing in the morning. I no longer knew how to co-ordinate colours or styles. I finally managed to work out a few simple sets of clothing, which I alternated from day to day, and the rest of my wardrobe just sat and stared at me.

I will never forget the feeling of despair as I leaned against the pantry door one day, wondering what all the things were, and how to use any of them. During this period I actually forgot how to do the most basic things such as boiling an egg and, some years later, had to refer to a basic cook book to re-learn the simple skills usually taken for granted.

I felt that I was in a different dimension or time zone. When my children reached out to me for simple advice, I found it difficult to interpret what they were saying, let alone find an answer. Their words seemed to be coming to me over a wide chasm, taking such a long time to reach me, and what I heard had no meaning.

Everyone, even my children, seemed to be in another world beyond my reach. I couldn't see them clearly, even when standing close by. At times I had trouble recognising them. It was as though they were people I used to know a long time ago. If they touched me, I couldn't really feel the touch. They could never break through the invisible wall that always seemed to surround me.

At this stage my speech was low and monotonous, with long pauses before answering. With some people, however, the processes are speeded up. Many people pace, wring their hands, or pull at their hair or clothing. This slowing down or speeding up is known as psychomotor retardation or agitation.

For a long time now, I had been unable to feel any normal emotions. No matter how hard anyone tried to show their love for me, I no longer knew how to respond. I dimly remembered that, somewhere in my past, I had experienced love, but now something was blocking my capacity to love, my ability to understand the feeling of love. Love was a meaningless word. And just as there was no love, equally there was no annoyance or anger, enthusiasm or warmth, humour, or pride in any accomplishments.

I was alone. Even my God seemed to have left me to do battle on my own. Spiritually I had been stripped bare, left dry and parched, and I decided that God was testing my strength just as Jesus was tested for forty days in the desert. I used to be very spiritual, going to church every Sunday, and had a faith that sustained me through all sorts of trials. But now I felt nothing – nothing at all. It was as though my soul had died along with my mind.

My deepest roots were embedded in Catholicism, and if these roots were to be sustained through life and death, then I must one day turn back to the Church. I sensed that my spiritual life must be closely interwoven with every other aspect of my life, like warp and weft, if I were to have peace of mind, but these thoughts were still the thoughts of a tired, hollow person, too tired and bound in pain to be able to open my mind and heart to the Church. Like family and friends, the Church would have to remain at a distance until my mind was healthy again.

Had I been able to feel anger, I would certainly have been angry that my mind had been taken away from me at this time, because it is the only tool we have to help us overcome illness and adversity. I had not succumbed to fear or despair following my brush with cancer because I had my mind, which was strong and healthy, and it carried me through with equanimity and peace. But this time I had nothing to fight with.

This fact is not very well understood by many people, who think the sick mind should still be able to produce the positive thoughts needed to get on with life. They do not realise that, bit by bit, the power of thought itself is removed. Telling a severely depressed person to 'snap out of it' is like telling a person who has broken legs to get up and walk.

During this episode, thoughts of death constantly filled my mind, like the hounds of Hell. There seemed no other answer, no way of escaping. Every object I saw, whether at home, at work, or along the road or street, became an object to procure my death. But because I had suffered so much already, I did not want to end up with a botched suicide attempt, so I did nothing. I still had memories of an unsympathetic hospital staff being angry after pumping my stomach following the overdose of pills when I was a teenager. I wasn't about to repeat such an incident. But death became a real obsession nonetheless.

I think it would be impossible to endure such a depressive episode without a psychiatrist, not just for the medication, but for the support and comfort he or she is able to give. If I remembered nothing else, I remembered the dates of my visits to my doctor. He was the epicentre of my existence and I clung to him fiercely, knowing that without him I would not survive.

That episode then lifted to a large degree, but it haunted me for a long time because I did not think I could withstand another onslaught like that. In August 1989, however, there was a sharp increase in the severity of anxiety and panic attacks, and I was no longer able to cope with them, even with added amounts of Valium. I became over-sensitive to everything around me – noise, light, people, crowded rooms, elevators, heights, open spaces, enclosed spaces. I was afraid of my own shadow. My physical and emotional reactions became exaggerated to the point where I often recoiled in terror if I stepped into the shadow of a tree as I walked along the footpath, and left badly shaken by the searing flash of panic.

Dr W. prescribed an anti-anxiety medication called Xanax. It is roughly ten times more potent than Valium, but works in a different way. Whereas Valium takes about thirty minutes to start working, and works over a long period of time, Xanax brings more instant relief, but its life-span is shorter.

It certainly did what it was supposed to. I could pop one before going out in the car in the morning, and the electric currents charging through my body would soon slow down. The only problem was the effects didn't last long enough, and in between doses I would still be a mess. I tried to persevere with the prescribed dosages, but found myself taking a Valium here and there just to top it up, to get me through the day. In no time at all I was taking eight to ten 5mg Valium a day as well as a number of the powerful Xanax.

The panic attacks increased and intensified with such ferocity that I quickly became immobilised the moment I left the comfort of my home. So, even though the depression had lifted somewhat at that stage, the anxiety took over to fill the gap. Again I was having to deal with both, and I just couldn't do it any more. Even on the days when I considered myself to be close to normal mood, I always felt a fragility of mind and body.

Finally, in September 1989 I was admitted to hospital for ten days – a psychiatric ward in a private hospital. At this stage I was so worn down by the persistence and severity of the illness that I even willingly agreed to another trial of Sinequan.

No sooner was I released from hospital than I swung into a high, spending huge sums of money in just a few days. I seemed to have a better understanding this time that perhaps my doctor should know about my spending habits. I visited Dr W. almost immediately and he arranged for me to be re-admitted to hospital with a change in medication, to protect the family finances from my uncontrolled spending, and to bring me down from my 'high'.

So I found myself back in hospital, out of harm's way where I was taken off the Valium by substituting clonazepam (Rivotril), an anti-convulsant which is also used to bring patients down from a 'high'.

For me, being high was wonderful at that time, because I felt so vivacious, so energetic. It was like being released from prison. My mind was my own again (or so I thought), and I was free to live and love. During this period, apart from my over-spending and general euphoric mood, my libido was heightened and there were periods when I seemed to be babbling over-excitedly and far too quickly. I also experienced an enormous burst of creativity. I wrote reams and reams of poetry, something which I had not done in many years. I didn't have much need for sleep, so day and night were both mine.

With a change in medication, the high mood settled down to a large extent, but from that moment until the end of the year, there were persistent small highs overriding my normal or depressed mood.

Meanwhile my debts kept mounting. When it comes to spending money the manic person sees a special need for everything purchased. He or she may invest money in a risky business venture with no sense of the consequence of these actions, and can very easily bring about financial ruin.

There are many agonising hours and sinking stomachs for the manic person following an episode where bizarre or embarrassing events have taken place, when the only explanation is 'I was crazy', and you wonder what on earth people around you must be thinking. Beth, forty-nine, writes of her most recent manic episode:

I was unaware at the time, but my mood was going up and down and then up again. I said we should go interstate to see if there was any work – we'd already gone elsewhere interstate a short time earlier. We took off, but came back in ten days' time and Jim could not understand why we had not looked around.

Then we were off to Western Australia. 'Let's buy a house there, away from all my memories,' I said. Jim thought this was a great idea. So we bought a house and came here just before Christmas. By now I was buying everything in sight, even a computer. About the middle of February I took a look at the bank statement and saw that I had spent $6000 in about six days. That was the downward trigger. I soon realised that I wanted to be back near my family, and things which were familiar.

But we were trapped because the house we had bought needed renovating completely before we could even try to sell it. This was the most dreadful time, the realisation that I had initiated these actions. It was about this time that I went into hospital and Jim began the 'doing up' process in earnest. Six months later I had recovered from the depression, made a few friends, and we were waiting to sell the house.

Time marched on for me, and 1989 was drawing to a close when I again became very depressed. The rate and content of my thoughts had slowed down again to almost a standstill, and I had very poor co-ordination. I was always visibly shaking, although I'm sure the latter was at least partly due to the effects of medication. I was guilt-ridden, and it centred largely around the fact that I was such a poor mother, wife and home-maker.

For a time I tried working with my guilt. Why should I feel guilty? Did I ask for this illness? Was I ever lazy, neglectful, irresponsible? I have always tried to be the perfect wife and mother. That option had been taken away from me through no fault of my own, so I should refuse to feel guilty. Perhaps the very essence of why I have been afflicted will prove to be learning how to relinquish control, to humble myself, to increase patience. I decided that, whatever happened, I would accept my illness and try to work through whatever it brought to me. When I talk of accepting my illness, I mean just that and no more. I do not mean resigning myself to it, or giving in, which is the way some people might interpret the remark.

In many ways this bout was not nearly as bad as the previous one, but because I was working, I was more painfully aware of my limitations and suffered great humiliations. I should not have been at work. I was nothing but a hindrance, but I struggled on, knowing that I must try to keep my job at any cost. One day merged into the next as though time did not exist, and I think the only thing that kept me going was the thought of a five-week break at Christmas time.

The two men I worked with did not know about my illness, and I had only started working there in the May of that year. One of these kind men completely took over my job during that period, as well as doing his own work. He had to watch my every move in case I bungled the few simple tasks that I tackled. I could not be trusted to do anything well, no matter how simple the task, even answering the telephone.

I was still suffering from the insomnia that accompanied all my bouts of depression, and my body clock was very regular, waking me around four every morning. I would lie there, agonising over the previous day's events, tormented by every word I had said, everything I had done, haunted by the knowing looks. Then I would turn back to childhood, searching for a reason for my being this way, but all I came up with was a myriad of bad thoughts and misdeeds, and I magnified everything out of all proportion until I knew I was worthless and I hated myself in the worst possible way. Then I turned to the day to come, which I always dreaded, knowing the whole process would repeat itself.

Yet, with all the pain of the depression, there were still overriding highs throughout much of it, times when I would create, socialise, and exude a great personality which almost belied the undercurrent of discontent and misery.

It was around this time that I discovered a book on manic-depression at the local library – the first one I'd come across – and I devoured it. The book is titled *Overcoming Depression* by Dimitri F. Papolos, MD, and Janice Papolos, and should be on the bookshelf of any home where this illness exists.

Towards the end of 1989 I again swung into a high. This time I decided to do something about my appearance because I was overweight and my hair was streaked with heavy bands of grey. I saw my hairdresser, then started dieting, determined to improve my self-image. A week later, on a routine visit to my dentist, I found a person completely sympathetic to my dilemma. He saw another way of improving my image, suggesting that he put overlays onto my front teeth which were badly discoloured and ground down. I did not need any convincing. When the work was completed, I walked out of his surgery with a confidence I had not thought possible. Beauty is not just the physical aspect, of course, but there is no doubt that the image in the mirror makes an enormous difference.

So, having been almost completely 'made-over', I decided to buy some new clothes. It was an exciting time and I barely slept that night. The following day, full of exuberance, I drove to my favourite shopping area. I did the rounds of the shops, elated, confident, and full of energy. As I laughed and chatted with salespeople, I was aware that my happy disposition was drawing attention. It was a good feeling to know that I was normal again and that my mood could affect other people's lives and make their day happier too.

Just as I was finishing off my shopping I ran into an old friend, and we stopped off for a chat and a drink. That was a Saturday, and somehow the chat and drink merged into the following day without my being quite aware of it. The rest of the weekend remains hazy in my mind.

What I do recall is spending most of the Monday plunged into depression, barely able to stumble through a dark day at work. Later that day, I opened the boot of the car. It was full of shopping bags. I actually looked at them wondering who on earth they belonged to and why they were there.

Fleeting images started emerging of the shops, the car park, the hotel, and the evening with friends. In my depressed state the guilt of this discovery darkened my mood even further. To make matters worse, I was not at all interested in any of the clothing, which was totally unsuitable. Years later, much of it went to charity without ever having been worn.

I merely existed for what remained of that year. George's mother had been very ill and she was hospitalised towards the end of the year, passing away in December. My state of mind made it impossible to grieve properly once she was gone. I just seemed aware of an added dimension of emptiness caused by the loss.

I remember when we sat with her during her last hours, talking but not knowing whether she could hear. Her flesh was a cold reminder that this moment awaits us all, the moment when the invisible soul, the spirit that makes each of us so unique, flees this life, leaving only the shell behind. I thought a lot about the body and the soul at that time, and decided that the shell retains its beauty even in death, because it has been the medium by which we made contact with the essence contained in the soul and the mind. The myriad of deep lines etched into her dear face told not only her age, but the story of her life – the laughter, warmth, hardships and strengths. Her eyes, when opened, had revealed the quickness of her mind and all her emotions, but her mouth, even while closed forever, still showed the courage and wisdom of a lifetime.

I knew I had lost a good and wise friend, one who would do anything for her family, and I knew that the void created by her passing could never be filled. I ached with the pain of this new dimension of emptiness, but still I was unable to grieve as I wanted to, as I knew I should. I could only hope that I would be returned to reality in time to mourn her passing with real tears, real emotion.

1990

By 1990 my illness had put an enormous strain on our marriage and family life in general, so George and I packed our bags and set out for Apollo Bay. Because of my enthusiasm and apparent 'sanity' following the depression in late 1989, George was very optimistic about our relationship. I was so convinced that I was normal again and so imbued with the spirit of love and affection (brought about by the high mood) that the horizons looked bright once more. The bubble was to burst later on, when we both realised that I was not the person we had thought I was during that holiday.

Unaware as we were of what was ahead, the short holiday was a wonderful time for both of us. There were quiet, brisk walks along the beach enjoying the wet sand underfoot and the wind ruffling our hair – both of which I found to be quite sensuous – watching beach cricket, or just looking at the seagulls. In fact, we spent more time watching life going on around us than we did participating. There were romantic nights in our little house, high on the hill beyond the nearby township of Morengo. The farmhouses in the valley below and the nearby townships were a vast panorama through our windowed wall, with the distant waters of the ocean completing the picture. Perched so high above the valley, we were a part of any storms that passed through, and we watched lightning streaking down into the valley, and sheets of rain drifting slowly and majestically across the vast sleepy hollow.

I spent days at a time writing poetry, which should have told me something about the state of my mind. George accepted me as I was, just happy that I was so enthused about life, not wanting to think about mental illness for a brief spell.

Soon after returning home, my moods became erratic, swinging backwards and forwards from high to low, until they smoothed out to a low-grade depression by the end of February. These problems were compounded by the fact that I was coming off clonazepam, and the withdrawal caused acute anxiety, and even hallucinations when I had finally finished with them.

The low-grade depression continued, but with overriding high symptoms, and the occasional day where I was low enough to feel suicidal. I then experienced an out-and-out high, a manic phase, during which I embarrassed myself by telling very risque jokes inappropriately, and dominating conversations loudly and aggressively. Many different ideas were popping into my head at a great pace, but I could not get them out quickly enough, so they came out in bits and pieces, almost staccato style. I had to resort to Valium that night to still the frenzy in my mind.

During a manic episode speech is very striking – what is called a push of words, or pressure of speech. The voice becomes loud and intense, with an insistence that allows no interruption from anyone, and words are spoken rapidly. In hypomania, this apparent enthusiasm can be quite appealing, but as the person soars closer to mania, thoughts begin racing and speech moves too quickly from topic to topic, leaving sentences uncompleted. Unfortunately, the seemingly inexhaustible mood disintegrates, often abruptly, into irritability and anger, leaving others bewildered by the incoherent speech and change of mood. The person may then spiral down into a deep depression.

The high affected my work and my relationships with some of my co-workers. During this particular episode I remember firing commands at my boss in an exuberant but aggressive manner, and I noticed him backing off, frowning and looking somewhat bewildered.

My chaotic thoughts were reflected in my work. I would start one job, then when I'd barely got it moving I'd think of another related job and start that. Then moments later I'd think of another, then another, then another, and start them all, till I had a mountain of paperwork on my desk, paper in the typewriter, but nothing achieved. During this period I was constantly out socialising at night, because I didn't need sleep and was filled with both an unstoppable exuberance and the need to keep moving, to go, go, go, mentally and physically. There was a burning need to be with people, laughing, dancing and drinking.

Many people turn to drugs or alcohol for relief from all the excitement, restlessness and agitation of a manic episode. Unfortunately this can also bring the added problems of dependency.

There are some who experience all of the effects described, but also continue to experience paranoia, grandiose delusions or hallucinations. They may have visions or hear voices. They might believe they have a special relationship to God or a special mission to save their country, and indeed might set about carrying out that important mission. Patty Duke Austin was one such person. She heard voices through the radio that told her that someone was taking over the White House and that she could be of assistance. Suddenly she flew into action, ringing people, and taking off instantly for Washington. Then, when she arrived there, the house of cards began to fall and she realised that her behaviour was not normal. Others, such as Beth and Marike, have found themselves in equally bizarre situations. Beth tells us:

> I think I can help a lot of people – for short periods I have even thought I could be Jesus Christ. This was very frightening and I did not tell anyone.

Marike, thirty-one, believed she was the 'Second Eve' and that she had come into the world to fix up the mess.

> This I did by chanting rhymes to lift curses from all countries in the world. I also did many other bizarre things associated with this: ritual cleansings, the writing of Hebrew prophecies and so on. With red texta I wrote symbolic prophecies in circular-style mirror-writing on the walls of my house. I was elated. I did not eat or sleep, except for a few hours on Tuesday, until the following Saturday night, when neighbours put me in an ambulance for hospital. When I heard my neighbours trying to break into the house I thought they were coming to murder me.

Jane Fonda will never know how much she helped me during some of those awful times. I felt so vital, alive and vibrant following the depressions, and often an aerobics workout at one in the morning to a Jane Fonda video was the only way to burn off the excess energy. Then I would sit down to a few hours of poetry writing.

It was so painful, however, when I left the high mood behind to discover I was not invincible, had no energy to exercise, and would never write a book of poetry. I was, in fact, nothing; a mere worm in the overall scheme of existence, a worm that no one would even care to know. I would then slip back, exhausted, into my depression.

Very passionate but short-lived interests are common when one's mood is elevated, and were quite pronounced with me during a high because of my nature, so determined and single-minded when pursuing any course of action. So when I decided early in the year to take up guitar lessons, it turned out to be something of an 'obsession'. I knew that there were great things in store for me – eventually I would be brilliant. I bought an electric guitar, amp and all accessories and started lessons. My future was so clear and exciting, and there was never any doubt in my mind. I also took up taekwondo with the same initial passion. I could definitely see myself as a black belt and I thought the benefits would be enormous, physically and mentally; after doing a few classes I was even more convinced. I thrived on the concentration and self-discipline required, and felt it was helping my illness enormously. But, after a few months, I became too ill to continue and realised that the whole idea was merely symptomatic of being high.

Toilet paper became another of my pet obsessions that year. It had to be apricot-coloured, and a particular brand, although if that brand wasn't available I would reluctantly settle for a second. If neither brand was on the shelves I would stand staring in disbelief for ages, comb the shelves, looking behind mountains of rolls in the hope that I would find my special paper. I would even go to another supermarket, because I had a terrible fear that something bad would happen in my life if I did not have my apricot-coloured paper. The wrong paper represented a lack of safety in my life in much the same way as when I was constantly checking the knobs on the kitchen stove or the dials on the gas heaters.

In May the panic attacks started again. I was constantly in a state of anxiety, or irritable and aggressive in my mixed state, sleeping only two to five hours per night. The higher I became the more the little motor inside me kept revving up, making me extremely restless, unable to be still. I felt I was losing control and began drinking more often, in an effort to drown out the pain. It was not long before I was back on the Valium and Xanax in a search for oblivion.

At this time I tried acupuncture for the relentless panic attacks, but it was not successful and I had to battle on, continuing with larger quantities of Xanax and Valium.

Around this time I met another new group of friends – kind, understanding people who accepted me just as I was, never questioning, never judgmental. They watched me popping pill after pill with shaking hands, saw my erratic driving, and watched my crazy moods, never saying a word. They just opened their hearts and took me in. These new friends knew nothing about my past so they were not in a position to make any comparisons between past and present. I could be just me. I would often stay overnight with one couple. If I had an irresistible urge to be unusually sociable, or if I needed to drown out my pain, they would always have a hearty meal ready for me and I would eat, drink and chat until I was happy and comfortable. Then there would be a bed ready for me because I was usually unable to drive home.

Other friends stood by me too, but my point is that it was also necessary to have friends who knew nothing about me, or my past, with whom I could relax.

Then September offered me the opportunity of a lifetime – a trip to Manila with some of my new Filipino friends. I certainly had a wonderful holiday, but it did nothing for my health. Before I left Australia I had been warned by Dr W. to keep up my daily fluid intake and to take a small pinch of salt from time to time to prevent fluid loss and the possibility of resultant Lithium toxicity. Being somewhat removed from reality, I was unable to heed the doctor's words, which were left floating on the air.

I came to realise later that I was on a high from the time I arrived in Manila, but I had thought I was merely 'spaced out', or even normal. It seems a true sign of mental illness – of this illness at least – that we think we are normal when we are not.

From the moment I arrived, I perspired profusely, losing a lot of fluid. At the same time I was suffering from premenstrual tension, usually caused by fluid retention, so I started taking my usual diuretic, Chlotride, as soon as I was settled in the house. I then began losing large volumes of fluid without having the slightest realisation of what harm I was doing to myself.

Within twenty-four hours I started menstruating, and during the following twenty-four vomiting and diarrhoea began. I rummaged around in my medicine chest and found some Lomotil, the antidiarrhoea tablets I'd brought with me, and started taking them, together with some antibiotics I'd brought for emergencies. These had been prescribed by a general practitioner in case I should develop 'Manila belly'. By this time I was losing an enormous amount of fluid, and obviously my Lithium levels were rising. Eventually the vomiting and diarrhoea subsided but were soon followed by a large painful swelling in the left foot. Blood tests showed this to be gout, a condition I've never experienced either before or since. It had developed as a result of my lack of care for my health.

Not being of very sound mind, I quite forgot to tell the Manila doctor about all the medication I was taking at the time. I'm sure she would have been interested to know that I was taking Valium, Xanax, Lithium and antibiotics, and also Lomotil and diuretics. So, quite unaware of all or most of this, she started me on a course of anti-inflammatory tablets and ointment. The tablets no doubt helped the gout, but would also have been increasing the blood levels of Lithium, which Voltaren has been known to do.

Throw into this hotchpotch of medications my daily use of Ventolin for an allergic wheeze, and the result was one very dangerous explosive cocktail. The process of Lithium toxicity had well and truly begun, only I was too spaced out to remember Dr W.'s instructions or to have any comprehension of what was happening to me. I was mentally confused.

I continued on my merry-making way, eating what my upset tummy would allow and drinking beer and whisky to combat the heat – but no water. Very soon my whole body trembled and shook violently and unremittingly to the point where I could barely stand, let alone walk up or down the one small step leading into the house, without assistance. My friends commented on my twitching muscles, failing memory and general frailty, but somehow I managed to retain a bizarre kind of zest for life.

Before I left Manila, the best food and drinks were brought in, and many guests arrived to say farewell. I returned alone to Australia and was delayed in customs for about three hours for not declaring certain goods I had brought into the country for friends. I was really in no condition mentally to fill out even the most basic of forms, and so unknowingly made a false declaration.

George met me at the airport, worried about the delay, and his mouth dropped as he saw my greyish pallor. I went straight to work from the airport, two days late, but was sent home again. My legs could barely support me; my whole body shook uncontrollably.

I was asked to discontinue the Lithium at that time, and was happy not to take it for the rest of the year. From time to time since I had first started taking it I had noticed co-ordination problems and trembling hands or leg muscles which I thought could result from Lithium, and I hoped a break from the medication would tell the story.

Miraculously my mood levelled out and remained fairly stable from then until December. I even managed to withdraw from Xanax. The small highs that I experienced were easy to manage and did not interfere too much with my daily living. I tried to include George in my life during some small highs, inviting him to come with me to a few suburban pubs to listen to the bands. What I chose was not his cup of tea – nor usually mine – but he came along once anyway in an effort to please me.

I then had to knuckle down and pay off the new load of debts incurred from my trip. I did not realise then how deeply in debt I would be, and for how long, although I had by now become accustomed to a large proportion of my wages going each week to the banks and institutions that catered for my excesses.

1991

Sweet memories ripple the surface
Of my discontent,
And I dream a while
of days gone by
When love touched my heart
For a moment in time.

Love cared for me then
With tender words
and thoughtful ways,
Reaching into my heart
To shape my weakness
into strength.

Then love slipped away
Like the shifting sands
And my cry was lost
On a heartless wind.

But the memories remain,
And once in a while
Ripple the surface
Of my discontent.

I wrote this short poem as I was slipping into depression again early in 1991. Shortly after this George and I decided to end our marriage – after twenty-three years. It was a very painful time for the whole family. We both saw our solicitors, who mapped out a form of property settlement, but we were unable to proceed with it because the housing market was so low. The estate agents advised us to stay put for another year if possible until the market lifted.

Faced with this dilemma, we decided that perhaps we could stay under the one roof, but live our own separate lives, just for twelve months or so until the housing market picked up. It would also give us a breathing space in which to give the matter some deeper thought. But I was feeling enormously stressed and decided to leave home for a while. I felt a great need to be alone. At the time I was unable to relate well to anyone around me. My depression was not severe, but certainly sufficient to colour my reactions to my problems, and my anxiety was just high enough to make me feel that I was 'going crazy' and might flip out completely. I needed solitude to think about my problems and where my life was headed. I often found that solitude suited me. I moved only to the next suburb, because I wanted to keep up contact with the family and the household.

I particularly worried about the effect all the upheaval was having on the girls. I agonised over their reactions. Would they think I had deserted them? Would they understand that I really was sick? Would they be confused? I felt so sad, for them and for what was happening to us all.

One of the girls reacted noticeably by withdrawing and I knew she had pronounced judgment on me. It was understandable considering her age and what she had already been through with my illness, but my heart ached for her. Oscar Wilde said: 'Children begin by loving their parents. After a time they judge them. Rarely, if ever, do they forgive them.' I hoped that mine would understand and forgive me.

Later in the year, when I was feeling particularly low, Natalie said, quite matter-of-factly, 'Don't worry Mum, you'll be on a high again soon and everything will be OK.' She seemed to take my fears with such equanimity.

I often spent time by the beach reading or pondering on my situation. I was trying to put my illness and my life in general into proper perspective. I could feel the depression worsening, but I told myself that none could be as bad as the previous ones. Not any more. I worked on my optimism, convincing myself that this present mood was just a 'shadow of the Beast' and no one is afraid of shadows.

I used every positive strategy I knew to carry on in the right spirit, and certainly for a while anyway, my new-found solitude helped. There were no noises, apart from the ticking of the clock, or occasionally the TV. There were no people, and only a rare telephone call, so I was able to work on helping myself.

To combat my anxiety and work on my self-esteem, I turned again to books recommended by my plastic surgeon in 1989: *Psycho-Cybernetics* and *The Magic Power of Self-Image Psychology* by Maxwell Maltz, MD, FICS. In these books he shows us how to change the self-image and thereby the personality and behaviour by using self-image psychology. Imagery plays an important part, pictures being more impressive to our automatic mechanism than words, and I was very interested in following through with two pictures that he suggests we form in our mind: 'building yourself a quiet room in your mind', and 'forming a new picture of yourself as you would like to be, as you like yourself'.

The second picture is self-explanatory, but in relation to the first picture he quotes Marcus Aurelius:

> Men seek retreats for themselves: houses in the country, seashores and mountains; and thou too art wont to desire such things very much. But this is altogether a mark of the most common sort of men, for it is in thy power whenever thou shalt choose to retire into thyself. For nowhere, either with more quiet or more freedom from trouble, does a man retire than into his own soul, particularly when he has within him such thoughts that by looking into them he is immediately in perfect tranquility; and I affirm that tranquility is nothing else than the good ordering of the mind. Constantly then give to thyself this retreat, and renew thyself … (*Meditations of Marcus Aurelius*, translated by George Long, Mount Vernon, NY, Peter Pauper Press)

Dr Maltz tells us how to build a quiet room within, in the imagination, in order to depressurise ourselves. Then, whenever there are a few moments in the day between appointments, or whenever tension is mounting, we can retire into our 'quiet room', leaving our worries behind, giving the nervous system the recuperation and protection it needs.

At times in the past, retreating into my private 'room' had been very beneficial, but I knew too that it became useless once depression took a firm hold. Dr W. was absolutely right when he said 'a person cannot be reached in severe depression'. There comes a point when you are lost to everything and everyone.

Sometimes my mind would be completely emptied of troublesome thoughts whilst in my room, which I easily remembered in every detail, but at other times I would use it to calmly work out a problem. The process was very helpful, but there was nothing I could do to halt the progress of this episode of depression, and by the end of February my strategies no longer worked.

Decision-making again became an impossibility as the black cloud descended, blanketing my world. One day, whilst still living away from home, I went to the supermarket. I stood in the aisle, staring at the endless array on the shelves, confused and powerless to decide. I walked away with nothing, full of guilt and self-loathing.

I drove to a nearby shopping centre and spent the money set aside for that week's bills on clothes, putting others on lay-by. I was used to spending thousands when I was high, but this was something new: I felt *nothing*, just a flat nothing.

The solitude was working against me now. At night the house seemed to be closing in on me. I wanted to scream with all my might, to burst through the walls to the fresh air outside. But I was too frightened to open any doors or windows. So I slept, with the light on, wishing the telephone would ring to bring me back to reality.

I recommenced Lithium on 10 February, and was now on a daily dosage of 1250mg. This was producing the side effects of nausea, dizziness, and trembling of the hands and legs, so the dosage was reduced to 1000mg. By now I was again prepared to talk about taking anti-depressants, recognising that the depression might not lift without further help. Because I had taken no tranquillisers for well over a month, and no other medications for an even longer period, I could now separate the effects of the illness and the medication, and gain a better understanding of my depression.

I was feeling quite removed from reality most of the time, unable to move beyond the front door, and I realised that I could no longer cope alone. Moving back home was the best thing I could have done. In fact it was the only thing. Once I had settled in again, our family life very soon continued on in the same old way. The girls were obviously very happy that things were 'back to normal' again, and it was a blessing to see them relieved of that stress.

By Easter I was still depressed, dredging up things from the past that now caused unbearable pain. They were usually trivial incidents that no one else would have remembered, but my mind often returned to these obscure moments in time, and made them into something of deep shame.

I happened to be standing at the kitchen sink during one such moment of recollection, separating grains of freshly cooked rice in an old yellow colander. My thoughts had been travelling back to a time early in my marriage when my parents were visiting us. I had just cooked dinner, and pulled out my new yellow colander to drain the vegetables. Unfortunately my mother dared to suggest that the colander was not suitable.

'It's good enough,' I snapped quickly.

Tears flowed freely now as I pictured the hurt I must have caused my kind, gentle mother. And later I would probably cry and feel guilty because I had let the rice go cold.

The following day I was hanging on by barely a thread. The tension and fear were overpowering, and I was using diaphragm breathing as a means of trying to stave off the surge of hyperventilation attacks that were almost bringing me to a standstill. There were no paper bags in the house, so I made one out of butcher paper and kept it with me, breathing into it when I needed to. My control was not good and I thought a glass of burgundy that night might be helpful in preference to Valium, which I really needed.

The need to write something meaningful and pleasing was rising to just below the surface. I was sufficiently depressed that clear thought was impossible.

I was recording a new depression when the scars of the old had not yet healed, and I relived the pain through my pen. Thoughts of death, constantly on my mind of late, now engulfed me. I feared that I might take the final step should the depression gain a firmer hold and leave me without control.

But I finished that night well, as my journal notes: 'The burgundy has done its work well now, so I'll try to sleep. I'd love to add some levity to this diary, to clear the cobwebs away; maybe my humour will surface again, rise from the dead, so to speak.'

With my depression now quite severe again, I commenced a course of Prozac, a new antidepressant that was supposed to produce remarkable results without the unwanted side effects of other antidepressants. Prozac brought renewed hope for the future, and they actually suppressed my appetite. At $25 per week one would hope for the best, surely!

But after a couple of weeks I swung into a high. I awoke one morning thinking I was completely normal, feeling a new energy stirring deep inside, and promising to surge to the surface. Really believing that the Prozac had worked a miracle for me, I said a prayer of thanks for being restored to normal, and then raced round to an old friend and told her of my miracle. She looked a bit dubious when I told her I was hearing in three-D, but said that perhaps it seemed that way because I had been depressed for so long. Little did we both know.

Funnily enough, the following day's journal entry used the word 'euphoria' to describe those happy feelings, but still I did not recognise the fact that I was already quite high.

For the following few days, my journal speaks of 'such clarity of thought and such a rush of thoughts that my pen cannot keep up with my mind', the 'mixture of contentment and excitement', and the 'mountains of writing' I'd done, taking only two hours' sleep each night. On the fourth day the entry says 'I feel on the verge of high, but with depression hanging like a cloud over my head'.

This descended in a mighty swoop without any warning, no spiralling down, but plummeting like a rock thrown over a cliff. Neither was there any fuzzy head or grey fog this time. I was enshrouded in darkness of the worst kind, my mind heaving in the throes of all-consuming guilt and pain. Every wrong thought, word or deed in my whole life burst into my mind. They screamed and pounded unrelentingly, allowing me no other thought. I wanted to cry with shame, to cleanse myself, but I couldn't. I knew my family would all be better off without me. This time I knew what I had to do.

I lay for two days, unable even to lose my grief in sleep. Then, as suddenly as it had overtaken me, it lifted – not completely, but from zero to about 30 on the graph (see page 67). That was when I quite calmly made my suicide plans. I would hardly say I was of sound mind. There was no doubt I was still very ill and in a state of shock, because I felt completely numb. The worst attack ever had left me in a state of despair, robbing me of any hope for the future, neither for myself nor for my family.

My first step was to arrange for a new will to be drawn up, in readiness for my signature the next day. Then I gave serious thought to the method. I supposed that drugs were the cleanest way, but I did not know which would be best. I did not want to choke on my tongue, drown in my own vomit or, even worse, live and be brain-damaged. So, the following day I went to the local library, and said I was writing a piece for college on the relationship between drugs and suicide among young people. I asked for statistics and whatever other information was available. While an attendant took me round the shelves picking out books and sheets here and there, she kept staring at me, asking me questions.

Finally she raced out the back, emerging a few moments later with the librarian in charge who came and talked to me. What precisely was I looking for? And what exactly was the nature of my assignment? Could he help me with the statistics? He hovered nearby, watching discreetly over his shoulder from time to time. It turned out to be a fruitless exercise for me, and I ended up leaving with nothing helpful.

I managed to get a copy of *Mims*, the book doctors and pharmacists use for complete drug information. I studied it, photocopied what I needed, and knew I had what I wanted. I then signed my new will and went home to bed, exhausted. I spent another two days in bed, sleeping no more than a few hours each night, but too fatigued to move. My mood level had lifted to about 50 at this time. By the end of that period I had lost the urge to end my life, knowing that at least I would not have to despair and feel trapped in the next attack, because I could always opt out.

The following day my mood spiralled down again to 20. No matter how sick I had been in the past, this seemed to be the most vicious and debilitating attack I had experienced. I was seeing the Beast for what it really was. It had complete control, absolute power, and I was its little plaything.

I slept for twenty-six hours straight. The following four days were also spent in bed, with only irregular sleep, but I did emerge to shower and eat from time to time.

Dr W. concluded that the Prozac was obviously not working for me, so I started a course of Prothiaden, another antidepressant, which I stopped after one month, partly because of side effects and partly because it seemed to be doing nothing for me. I had also stopped the Lithium again at this stage because of trembling hands and muscle spasms in the legs, so I was taking no medication at all. The result remained to be seen.

Early in July, because of the great fluctuations between low and high, Dr W. decided to start me on Tegretol, which is an anticonvulsant, or anti-epileptic, drug. This, combined with Lithium, often has a very good effect with illnesses that are difficult to treat. Overall throughout July my mood was quite stable, and there was even one period where I felt it to be 100 per cent. I made the most of this to visit my parents in Albury – something they had been wanting me to do for a long time.

To go to Albury was a big breakthrough, and I was very much aware of this as I stood in the waiting area at Spencer Street railway station. I felt a sudden surge of excitement and an almost overwhelming nostalgia. For a brief moment I was young again, travelling between cities, amongst strangers, wondering who my travelling companions would be. But this time it was slightly different, this time there was a new element – trepidation.

The aroma of hot food wafted across to me and, although I did not expect to find gourmet food, the idea of breakfast was suddenly a good one. I bought a croissant, and headed for the platform. There was only one young man seated, and I shared the same bench, wondering why everyone else was standing. It didn't take long to realise that, at seven o'clock on a cold wintry morning, who in their right mind would want to sit on a chilly metal seat? After a while the young man turned to me, a pained smile on his face as he changed position. He knew I understood, and we both chuckled. 'I'm so bloody tired, I have to sit!' he moaned, rubbing the numbness away. It was only a brief exchange between two strangers, but the lighthearted encounter drew me back to reality for a moment, away from my apprehension. The time was not far off, I thought, when I would be strong enough to reach out more and more into the world around me.

The trip was comfortable, and I spent my time reading or sleeping, so the four hours passed quickly and with no claustrophobia, what's more. When the Albury station came into view the carriage quickly emptied as people milled around the doorways. Now it was my turn. I stepped out and peered to my left down the long platform where I expected my father to be. There were so many people it was difficult to pick anyone out. Suddenly he was there, seeming to emerge out of thin air, and my shoulders were soon cradled in the familiar warmth of his arm. Home. Home, at last. And in a short while, there was Mum waiting for us at the front door. She could hardly contain her happiness and excitement at seeing me after eighteen months. I realised then how much I must have hurt her by my absence – but such is the nature of the Beast. I couldn't stand there feeling guilty; I had to make the most of this time together, and keep looking ahead to a brighter future.

And things did pick up. When I returned from my trip, I enrolled in a St John Ambulance course for work, so that I could become the official First Aid person, and even with impaired concentration and memory, I obtained a Senior Level 2 Certificate. To other people, this was a real non-event, but to me it heralded great things to come.

When inevitably my mood lowered again I was finally so worn down that I felt the need to go to hospital for a while, just to have a rest, but a friend invited me to her home instead, offering to look after me for the weekend. So I sobbed my heart out to her on the Saturday and then spent the rest of the weekend in bed while she and her husband pottered around the flat, did their shopping, and cooked meals for me. I felt like an unprotected child needing lots of love and reassurance, and somehow they were able to give it to me.

I got through the week, but by the following weekend my body and mind were totally depleted of energy and I slept from Friday night until Sunday afternoon. By the next Friday I was in hospital for a few days' rest.

Hospital care provided me with the comforting knowledge that there was a qualified staff to look after me should I be unable to look after myself or become suicidal, caring staff to bring my meals and medication and check that I was feeling OK, or just to talk if that was what I needed. In hospital one does not feel a burden, because one is being cared for by paid staff.

By the end of the week after I went home I was bouncing like a rubber ball between angry excitement and flatness, with a drop of anxiety thrown in for good measure. I was either eating too much or not hungry at all — it came in waves. On the Saturday I went with a friend to a wonderful little deli in South Melbourne where we both loved to eat. I tried hard to talk but my mind was too slow to respond, my mood too flat. Sometimes I managed to feign some believable laughter — or so I thought — but my mind had trouble keeping up.

After about one and a half hours the conversation around us seemed to be getting louder and louder, closing in on me, but my friend's voice was growing more distant, fading away. I had to read her lips to know what she was saying. My head was swimming and I felt as though I were floundering in a tumultuous sea, unable to breathe. I tried to focus on my friend's face but found it difficult to concentrate. Suddenly, without warning, I stood up. I had to leave before I became caught up in a panic attack. As we drove home, I knew it was better for both of us that we had left when we did.

I can say with certainty that my life is never dull. October 1991 was a good example. I veered from a period of gay abandon, partying, drinking and spending lots of money, to a spot so low that I felt suicidal and had to ring Lifeline in the early hours of the morning. Thoughts of death took hold and flourished to the point where I feared I might attempt suicide if I were plunged any further into depression. I didn't want to take my life, but knew well that I might try. The person on the other end of the line had to work very hard that night to keep me focused on my two daughters and how much they love me and need me.

Thankfully November brought me a normal mood before the highs of December set in. Looking back, it seems that spring and summer have often brought on the most noticeable highs for me, the ones that cause the most distress and disruption in my life.

I remember one day early in that December when I felt so happy that I just had to talk to people. I flicked through my teledex and made a number of calls, anxious to tell people that I was back to normal again. It was so good for me to hear the pleasure in their voices when they remarked on how well and happy I sounded. I even rang one person I had not spoken to for about ten years. What I did not realise was that my mood was escalating very rapidly, and because I had an abundance of energy, I kept people on the phone for so long that they soon tired.

I expressed to George my need to gain some independence, to 'find myself'. This must have been a difficult pill for him to swallow, but his reply was calm. 'Let's just go on and see what happens,' he said. Perhaps he recognised the fact that I was high, even though I myself had not yet realised it. I stayed up working until two in the morning and planned exciting things to do. Of course, being up and busy twenty hours or more each day meant I was also smoking more, and the more frantically my thoughts raced the more I smoked – a very unhealthy situation.

But the most disturbing aspect was my insatiable need to socialise, drink and dance. The rhythm of the loud, fast rap music pulsated through my veins with an intensity I could not resist. All I wanted was to go wild on a disco dance floor, to be drunk on the beat of the music, and then to drink, and drink some more in gay abandon. There was an urgency in my need to socialise with new people, as well as to renew old friendships.

When my doctor suggested at this point that I was high, I was able to say 'no' with all sincerity. I had certainly considered the possibility but had to dismiss it because of a lack of many of the usual signs: I was not constantly telling jokes, dominating conversations, or continually laughing. Nor were my thoughts frenzied. Some of these symptoms might be present occasionally, but at other times my conversation was normal, even irritable. So, to my mind, that equated to normal mood fluctuations. I did give a lot of consideration to the restlessness, which I really could not understand, but I eventually concluded that, because I had been going through such a rough patch in my life, it was quite normal to develop a need for some independence, some freedom from my problems.

By the time I had been overcome by the urge to go to a disco, I realised that I had no suitable clothes. I raced out and bought four new outfits, complete with the appropriate jewellery for each. The cost was around $1000, on credit of course. This was quite a standard amount for me to spend in one day.

As I stood in the fitting room trying the clothes on, I questioned the necessity to buy four outfits, especially when I saw the look of amazement on the face of the saleswoman turn to glee. It had quickly become obvious to me that, in fact, four outfits would not be anywhere near enough for my new lifestyle. I would, however, be conservative this time.

It did cross my mind that this was another 'first' for me, another new experience, to be spending so much money when I was normal – very normal, in fact. I would even be happy to show George the clothes this time because he would be taking me dancing and would realise the necessity. He would be pleased to see me looking so good. In fact, when I thought about it, I would have to buy him some new shirts before I went home. He had nothing at all suitable for nightclubs and discos.

All in all, I was satisfied with the success of the day. Sure, it was a little extra on credit, but it would bring a lot of happiness into our lives and, under the circumstances, I did not feel I'd been extravagant at all.

Soon after that little spree I began my new lifestyle, but without George. I was out with women-friends, talking, laughing, drinking, and above all, not sleeping. It lasted only a matter of days, however, before my mood collapsed. Then I saw what had really happened to me, and I became very despondent, grieving over the loss of what I had thought was my return to normal life.

It was such a disappointment that I had not been able to recognise the elevated mood, that I had not listened to my doctor, and I decided there and then to once again put my credit cards out of sight. I asked George to remind me of this episode if I became so restless again. Unfortunately, the highs always came in a different guise and I always seemed unable to recognise them until it was too late.

Shortly after this, I was telling a friend how difficult it can be to recognise a high. She said, 'How are you now?' to which I replied, 'Terrific, fine, back to normal'. She roared laughing and said, 'How do you know? Are you sure you're not just a bit high?' We both roared, and I said, 'Who knows, who cares? I just feel good'. This loses a lot in the telling but it came hot on the heels of my telling her of the message I'd recently put on my aunt's seventieth birthday card:

'As you slide down the bannisters of life,
May the splinters go the other way.'
Luckily, my aunt has not lost her sense of humour!

1992

My first and probably most important decision in 1992 was to inform the two men I work with about my illness. Ultimately I had no choice because my concentration and memory were not what they should be; I did make mistakes, did forget. Usually they were minor, but this time I was being asked to remember an important incident which I was completely unable to recall. 'How could you not remember?' 'You must remember.' My boss was incredulous. He was right, of course. Anyone else would have remembered.

Talking about it was very upsetting, but once it was out in the open, both men were very understanding and, in the long run, it has made life easier for all of us. Of course, not everyone has an understanding boss, and the stigma attached to this illness still persists in many parts of the community.

Following this, I decided to do something positive to improve my general health and fitness. I joined a gym. At last I had a goal, a sense of purpose. I recalled the old saying 'a healthy mind in a healthy body' and hoped that my mental powers might increase as my physical fitness improved. This goal gave me the means to provide myself with regular challenges to meet, hurdles to overcome, and a way of improving my confidence and self-esteem. Every time I walked through the door of the gym I had won a battle. Every time I increased the weights or the number of repetitions, I had won another battle. But the depression worsened and I could no longer face extra exertion. I remember the feeling of defeat on my last attendance at gym, as I walked out the door.

Death had been following me around like a child seeking attention. This time I knew it was because all the signs of a lingering depressive episode were present and had been for the past week. Death always seemed the only way out, even though I didn't really want to die – not while I was relatively well, anyway. But I felt my tolerance level lowering quickly. At this stage the Tegretol was increased, and I immediately noticed the unpleasant side effect of nausea. I was also experiencing slight double vision.

I was filled with an immense nameless fear over the next few days. I had to sleep with the light on, propped up on pillows, and the days merged into one. The pressure inside my chest was intense, painful, as the muscles clenched into tight balls. If I lay flat, the anxiety welled up, I became phobic, and gasped for air. Often I would wake after a couple of hours, unable to go back to sleep. After a warm drink and a cigarette, I usually managed to drop off to sleep until around four o'clock when I would again awake, bombarded with my usual morning recriminations. I often felt able to drop off into useful sleep around seven, just about the time when I had to get up for work.

Again the Tegretol was increased, but this time my vision was very disturbed. I was seeing the whole room in two distinct images about thirty centimetres apart, and each image was like the undulations of ocean waves, so that I had to walk round with my eyes closed, or peering out of one eye, the lid barely opened because of nausea. I rang my pharmacist to see if this was a normal reaction. He thought it too severe to be considered normal, so I rang Dr W. who lowered the dosage. From then on it was a matter of making constant adjustments, slowly inching the dosage up to a point where it was effective but not high enough to produce such severe double vision.

The vision problem interfered with my job because using my eyes for close work made it worsen. A number of times I had to take twenty to thirty minutes off until the double or wavy vision subsided. Twice I had to go home early because I simply could not continue. I went to see an eye specialist who discovered that I had convergence insufficiency, where the muscles behind the eyes do not work together but pull against each other, a problem that I had had since birth. Until now, though, its minor effects had not caused any noticeable problems. It was the Tegretol that had exacerbated the condition.

Returning one day from the other side of town after visiting a friend who also suffered from depression, I looked at the crowded footpaths, wondering if a person existed who could understand and help me. Was there such a person in this mass of frail humanity? Life drove past me, walked alongside me, traffic lights changed, and changed again, but all I saw was a sea of troubled humanity making a futile attempt to find a happiness that didn't exist. It all seemed a waste of time.

On that unhappy note, I went home and settled down in front of the TV with a litre of icecream and a fistful of cigarettes: my trusty friends in time of need. At least my life had not been completely wasted that day, I thought dourly. At least my friend had benefited from my company. But my mood continued in the same vein, as my journal shows:

Life seems so futile somehow. We're a bunch of puny little creatures striving to make worthless dreams come true, all heading nowhere, falling down all over each other time and time again.

Friends and laughter have turned into ghosts and tears, the challenges into oppressive yokes. I have lost all control of myself, my life. I fought a good fight, but eventually it has become easier to give in. I no longer want friendship and laughter. It's so much less stressful to be alone, not having to try or to pretend.

I returned to the gym through that bout of depression, with great difficulty. Not only was the depression interfering with my energy levels, but an old problem reappeared to alarm me. It was rather like the odd skipped heartbeat that I had experienced earlier, only much more painful. An ECG done within the past few years had shown all to be normal, so I wasn't worried about my heart. I thought it was probably connected somehow with my medication or a symptom of anxiety.

This is an extract from my journal during that episode:

Monday being what it was, I crawled into my bed that night, knowing I wouldn't go to work the next day. It was too much of an effort putting on a cheerful face and having to cope with making even the smallest decision. I couldn't face the world, tied as I was to my guilt and despair. The guilt is all-consuming, dragging me down further and further into a world of darkness where I thrash wildly, cradling my grief. I'm all alone in a world where nobody can reach me, and there's no escape.

The guilt attacks in waves, like soldiers on the battlefield, determined to crush me. It takes me back to my childhood, and chastises me for all my wrongdoings …

Tuesday merges with Wednesday and I still haven't left my bed. I haven't showered or eaten, have only slept in the oblivion that Valium brings. I want to end it all, be free of the pain, and allow my family to live a peaceful life without me …

Now, on Wednesday afternoon, I'm awake, feeling a little better … I slowly ease myself out of the bed, sitting for a while on the edge. A wave of nausea surges into my throat and I have visions of it erupting all over the floor. My head feels light, empty, my hands shake, the trembling spreading quickly through my body and down my legs. As I stand up, my knees buckle slightly and I think I'm going to fall …

I take my nightie off, walking to the bathroom as if in a fog. The tiles are white, cold. At least they're not black like my inner world. I stand a while on the coldness, wondering what to do next. Do I turn the shower on? Or take my towel from its rail? The decision is too hard to make, so I reach for the towel without further thought and throw it on the tiles in front of the shower recess. At least I've made a move ... At least I am here in the shower, and not in my crumpled bed. It's a start.

Following that episode, I decided that being in bed for two days with a sick mind should be no different from being confined to bed for two days with the flu. It had taken a long time to reach that conclusion. Firstly I had to go through the stage of denial, then a very long period of gradual acceptance, to stop feeling sorry for myself, to realise that I was not the only one with this illness, and that it was really just an illness like any other. I tried very hard to maintain a positive attitude, to prove that mental illness need not preclude me from leading a relatively normal life.

But any sense of normality was difficult to attain, dogged as I was by illness and other passing health problems such as the shingles which erupted mid-year and lasted a few months. There were evenings when I would curl up on my couch, feeling physically as though I were pinned down under some enormous weight, crushed physically and mentally. It was too much of an effort even to open my eyes.

Dr Morison Tarrant, the Sydney psychiatrist quoted by Janet Hawley in 'The Darkness Within' (*Good Weekend*, 29 April 1995), speaks of the complete lack of physical energy experienced during his depression. He sums up and echoes the experiences of all of us who know severe depression:

> ... I was in complete slow mode, like a slow-motion movie. I had no energy, no interest, everything becomes a monumental effort, even to take a shower – my wife would put a chair in there as I didn't have the energy to stand. I saved up all my energy for the walk from the bed to the chair. I didn't have any other energy ... I had a startled response to everything; if the phone rang it was like an explosion and it took me half an hour to settle ... I could not will myself out of this illness any more than fly to the moon. Depression is not about a failure of will or moral strength, it's about one of the important functions of the brain not working properly ...

Dr Tarrant also points out the inability of people generally to understand the effects of severe depression, and expresses his anger that depressed people are generally thought to be lazy and lacking in moral fibre:

> ... The average lay person ... doesn't know that they don't know about the intricacies of biochemistry. They don't know that they don't know about the true nature of depression ... Depression is so common ... it's pathetic we haven't got around to teaching people in high school about it because we have such a high suicide rate among the young. Depression can kill you if you don't take it seriously.

Film-maker Jane Campion is quoted in the same article:

> Mum started to go into depression about the same time I was reaching adolescence ... and I remember feeling incredibly scornful about her. The usual lack of adolescent compassion ... I just hated the fact that she seemed to be hopeless at everything she tried to do.

> As I became older and able to show some compassion, I entered into her world too deeply and it really scared me ... I remember feeling the blackness she had developed through her depression just overpowering me too, and at those times I had to reject her and get away because I couldn't breathe. I couldn't see my own optimism any more. Depression is so seductive and her way of looking at the world seemed almost contagious, to the point that at one time I said, 'Look Mum, if you would really like to die and think you will be happier, I'll help you.'

> And she said to me, 'I don't want to die, I want to feel good about things.' And that was the turning point for me ...

Jane then introduced her mother to psychiatrists; she was eventually helped by having electroconvulsive therapy (ECT), and had been well for a year at the time of writing.

For the manic-depressive person, that lowest of low points can just as quickly be left behind as mania or hypomania takes over, particularly in the rapid cycler. Or, as with a mixed state, the depression can partially lift, and symptoms of hypomania can be experienced at the same time. This can be very confusing, troublesome and painful.

Following my last period of depression, I experienced this uncomfortable state, which has existed throughout my illness. It seemed to me that I had a split personality. The depressed side did not want to be social or even to eat, but there was another side ticking away at an enormous rate, trying to burst out. This side was frantically designing a new winter wardrobe, obsessed with the colour yellow, and anxious to be at the sewing machine. It pursued erotic fantasies with faceless men, and took me to dimly lit discos where I raged all night with unstoppable energy. A smaller part of me, clearly isolated, watched these two destructive forces battling for supremacy, seeing it all so clearly, and wanting them both to evaporate. The pain in my chest from tension was enormous, a gripping tension that threatened to erupt into a rush of uncontrollable energetic activity.

Leaving the mixed state behind, I slipped into depression. I constantly sought solitude, going out of my way to avoid people, becoming resentful and irritable when my private world was invaded. Most of the time I succeeded in being courteous, pleasant and patient, but I doubted that the smile reached my eyes very often. My self-loathing at this time often resulted in my not taking my medication. I would look at it with hatred and disgust, turning away, wishing it to hell.

I even showed impatience and hostility to strangers, and often found myself becoming very agitated, strumming my fingers on shop counters while waiting for change, anxious to be gone. In the car it was the same: I had to be on the move, hands clenching the wheel, constantly checking mirrors, anxious and impatient at the lights. This high side of my mixed state was showing up as hyperactivity and tension.

I backed out of several important social commitments around this time, and also a trip to Albury to visit my parents. I simply could not face the enormous strain of sitting through hours of polite conversation. It was generally a bit easier to muster a little patience with my family, because home has always been my haven. But the family unit appeared to me to be abnormal, heading towards some unknown disaster. I was projecting my general fears onto a family with the usual strengths and weaknesses.

There was a wonderful little interlude around this time when my mind cleared. Sounds, particularly in conversation, seemed so close and crisp, even sharp. The fog had visibly lifted, taking with it the hazy edges of sounds and shapes, and I was quite amazed at the difference. Sadly, those days are lost to the memory when the mood again takes a turn for the worse, as it did. I was so frightened, just wanting to blot everything out in sleep and then wake up normal and healthy again, knowing that everything I saw, touched, felt and thought was real. I did not know any more what emotions were normal, what thoughts valid. I felt disconnected from this world, out of focus, and everything around me looked and sounded hazy, as though they were not where they should be in time and space.

The remainder of that winter brought with it many different infections, an operation to relieve a stress-related medical condition, and ever-changing moods which fortunately did not fluctuate too far above or below the norm. The skies no longer looked so bleak because, although I was not completely well, I had definitely climbed to a higher rung of the ladder towards good health.

I now hoped to get on with the business of collating my copious notes taken over the past few years with a view to passing my knowledge on to others. I had toyed with the idea for a long time, knowing that my personal story could be beneficial. I kept up the journal entries with the book in mind, but there were so many times when I doubted my capabilities. Was it only my highs talking, telling me that I could produce a good book? Was my normal self actually capable? Certainly when I was on a downer I scrapped the idea altogether, firmly believing that I had grandiose ideas. But at other times I just knew I could do it. The actual structure of a book, researching and interviewing, were all matters of commonsense to me, and even with a modicum of talent plus the material I had available, it seemed a crime not to provide others with the knowledge I had gained.

I sounded out friends on the idea, particularly when I thought my mood was normal. When I told one very sensible friend of my doubts, she said, 'Oh, it's natural that you'll have doubts, but I know you can do it.'

'You don't think I'm crazy?' I asked.

She laughed. 'Of course you're crazy – but I still think you should write the book. I know you can do it.'

This friend had always been one to be trusted, so I kept on mulling over the idea, continued keeping my journal, and occasionally spent days at a time putting pieces of it together in some sort of cohesive form on the computer.

I knew by now that it was definitely a project I wanted to go ahead with, and thought I was capable of doing it justice. All it required was perseverence, instead of weaving complex webs of doubt in my mind.

It was not long, however, before spring heralded a frenzied high that lasted throughout much of my two weeks' vacation. This time I was driven not towards spending money or writing, but towards gardening.

During this time I was driven to create a whole new garden at the rear of our home. And it had to be an 'instant' creation, not to take seven days as with the creation of the world, although I was soon to discover that seven days was not enough, even for my small patch of land.

I had no rest during this episode, either physically or mentally. My thoughts were like a herd of wild horses thundering about in my head, racing first in one direction then another, then another, unable to be tamed. I needed to be physically active to obtain any relief from this mental agitation, and gardening provided a harmless release. The only damage done was the ultimate $1600 for material which I could ill afford, as I was still paying off credit card debts incurred during previous highs.

The evenings and nights were the most difficult periods to endure, as I was unable to remain still. On two nights I was out in the garden working in the rain after midnight, unable to find any relief from the frenzy in my mind. When I finally put my head on the pillow during that week, it was not to sleep but rather to decide in which direction every nail would be hammered the following day, how far into the wood each nail would be driven before being bent back to secure wire mesh to the fence, how deep each hole would be for each plant, remembering each individual weed that needed pulling, and in what order each job would be done. Then I would lie there urging the sun to rise quickly so that I could be busy again. If I slept two hours each night I was lucky.

(Two months later I realised that my chaotic thoughts were definitely reflected in the unco-ordinated appearance of two of the beds, and I had to set about achieving harmony and balance. More time, more work and more money.)

During my gardening frenzy I was busy planning how to do a family tree on my father's side. And I did not stop there. I planned our dinners for the following week, what I would wear in the garden next day, what other plants I would buy and from where, organised my finances – or lack of them – and dealt with a million other incidental thoughts that kept intruding. Each night was spent in the same manner. What distinguishes the thought process during a high like this is the frenzied way in which thoughts literally explode into the consciousness, eventually incoherent and unstructured. The mind is unable to deal with one thought at a time and follow it through – rather, the thoughts trip over each other, all vying for attention at the same time. I found, too, that the thoughts became loud, and I often heard them as voices chatting busily inside my head. It became very distressing, and I found myself reaching for Valium after four nights, to quell the agitation. Of course it had no effect, and the following night I doubled the dose, still with no effect.

That high episode was one of my most distressing to date, and Dr W. prescribed haloperidol (Serenace), a major tranquilliser used to bring people out of a manic episode, so that I should not have to suffer the same distress again. However, he believes that Lithium is generally the drug of choice in treating a manic-depressive illness such as mine, and the Serenace would only ever be used for short periods to bring my mood down quickly.

I returned to work after my 'holiday', feeling as though I'd been through the wringer. I was panicky and anxious, and work's little problems caused me great stress, although I tried to be relaxed and cheerful. But my moods continued to fluctuate daily from periods of hyperactivity to inaction, with a few glorious moments of relative calm. After one week my state of exhaustion forced me to take two days off, and I slept almost the whole period, utterly exhausted. During the second evening I still felt tired, physically and mentally, but there was a familiar buzz of activity starting up in my head. Suddenly I was aware that the answers to many previously puzzling thoughts and emotions were literally jumping into my mind with great clarity. It was like looking into a crystal ball, having answers appear without even having to ask the questions.

The restlessness and hyperactivity increased, and after going to bed, I found myself going downstairs again, wandering from room to room, smoking, straightening books and ornaments, writing, and wishing the house was full of people partying, so that I could drink and dance away my agitation. In fact, the the urge to put on a slinky dress and go partying was quite strong. I suddenly remembered the Serenace. Was it appropriate to take one now? I picked up the phone to ring the doctor, but I could not ring in the middle of the night.

I went back upstairs. Perched on the edge of the bed I looked at the bottle of Serenace and decided to go ahead. At around four o'clock I took another and lay down, wondering what was ahead before dawn. My head was still buzzing. I could hear millions of muffled voices somewhere in the background, whispering excitedly. My body felt like a wound-up toy soldier whose key is stuck, making the release of tension and stored energy impossible.

The next thing I remembered was the radio waking me at seven. I could still hear the flurry of voices, but they were more subdued, as though someone had turned the volume down. I felt that another couple of Serenace and another day in bed would have been very beneficial, but I started organising myself for the day ahead.

During the short period of relative stability that followed, I reflected on what I thought was a total change in personality. It seemed to me that the storm of the past five years had abated as suddenly as it had erupted, leaving me stranded, waif-like, on the pile of rubble left in its wake, faced with the task of salvaging and rebuilding.

Those years had conditioned me to the fact that I was completely under the control of my moods. And now, when it appeared that some control had been handed back to me for a while, I quickly discovered I did not have the confidence or necessary skills to take charge of my life.

Even when my mood seemed relatively normal I felt very flat. I knew that was often an effect of taking Lithium long-term. If so, would I have to learn to live life with the edge permanently taken off? If this was going to be 'normal' for me, then I would need professional help to rebuild the skills of communication and interaction, and regain and foster tolerance, patience, self-esteem and confidence.

I decided to reduce all my medication to the minimum dose, without my doctor's knowledge, to see if the flatness of mood eased. It was a risky step, and a mistake I would not make again. Certainly, the flatness eased. It was even followed by one glorious day of total peace and calm. Was this what it was like to be post-Lithium? No flatness, no heartache, no muffled voices, no urge to rage or spend. Just a stillness, a perfect calm, and a harmony of body and mind.

It did not, however, register that that day I had gone out and bought two CDs and $50 worth of car cleaning products. I cleaned the car inside and out for the first time in twelve months and went for a drive. After a while I noticed that the stillness I was experiencing now had an eerie quality to it – rather like the calm before the storm.

By bedtime, I was well aware that my mood was accelerating, that I was in fact high. I recommenced my medication, but I was still glad to have had that one perfect unforgettable day, no matter what the cost.

I had proved, though, that I do need my Lithium, that I do have an illness that cannot be denied, and requires daily medication. Theoretically I knew this all along, but sometimes we all feel the need to test ourselves, for various reasons such as anger, over-confidence, denial, or even because we're carrying too much weight as a side effect of one of the medications. But I have proved more than once that reducing or withdrawing medication without the doctor's approval ultimately results in a setback in recovery time. The moods, high or low, will come and go at their whim, and the medication is necessary to restore and/or maintain them at an acceptable level.

Serenace kept my high at an acceptable level for most of the remainder of the year. In fact, there were many days when I found the mood quite to my liking because it was just where I wanted it – at a level that provided high energy and lots of enthusiasm, but without the nastiness of frenzied thoughts. I was happy at work and mixing well.

On reflection, I could now see that the illness had not only changed its face quite dramatically in 1991 and 1992, but that the changes had been for the better. I decided that from now on I would be able to treat it not so much as an illness, but rather as an inextricable part of me, like a mole on my back perhaps, which sought no sympathy and no special attention other than monitoring, charts and medication, and little or no conversation about itself.

No doubt being slightly high helped me develop this attitude, but nonetheless it was the turning point where I felt, for the very first time, that I could accept the illness as my constant travelling companion, warts and all, until its time was up, that I could now step forward in a more positive manner.

The first step I took was to make an appointment with a cardiologist to have an ECG whilst on a treadmill, just to make sure there was nothing drastically wrong before I resumed my gym workouts. The appointment was made for February, and the gym agreed to hold my membership open until that time. With this in mind, 1993 loomed like a bright star on the horizon, and I eagerly anticipated Christmas for the first time in years.

Our family celebrations are held in Polish tradition on Christmas Eve, and this year started out like all others, hanging the wreaths and other decorations, decorating the tree and preparing the food, each doing his or her bit to help, and all of us looking forward to the evening meal and exchanging gifts.

We finally settled into our dinner amid laughter and merriment. It was a very special Christmas this year, and we all felt it – that special sense of togetherness and harmony that hadn't been present for the past five or so years, due to my illness in part, but also to the death of George's mother three years before. For myself this good feeling was partly because I was no longer surrounded by the fog of the past few years.

We were a complete family again, and the atmosphere of relaxed good cheer was noticeable as we chatted around the table. Tanya had returned after living away from home for the past six months. She was beautiful tonight; alive and bubbly, her skin clear and fresh, with the light catching the warm gold highlights in her hair. Natalie was also sparkling. For the first time she had been earning good money this year, and had gone out of her way to find gifts she knew we would all love. It seemed that this year everyone was determined to make Christmas memorable.

Then someone dropped a few thoughtless words. Something snapped inside me and I retaliated sharply. I think it was the depth of the feeling that helped me to recognise that this was not just the result of a few ill-chosen words, but was the anger and irritability of a mood swing.

At midnight I attended a local church for Mass, but found I had little patience for it. My mind kept wandering and I wanted to be on the move. When I finally went to bed, I was unable to sleep. I wanted to be up and busy, doing some charitable work. I decided that I must go to a soup kitchen or some other institution to offer my services for Christmas Day. I would have gone right then but I lay there impatiently until I saw four and then five o'clock. Shortly afterwards I drifted off to sleep and the next thing I knew it was mid-morning. I had awakened with a terribly heavy head and a body to match. A hangover could not have been much worse. I rolled over, dismayed, and shut the world out again.

Eventually I had to join the rest of the family because they were all preparing to leave on their various holidays, and so on. The heaviness lifted only slightly, and the irascible mood was still present. Very soon the wavering images of double vision were causing severe nausea. A little rest on the couch to quell this lasted on and off for three days, alternating between bed and couch, my head feeling hung-over, my libido becoming more and more insistent, and my nerves becoming more and more frazzled.

To make matters worse, I had become quite paranoid. I had experienced such extreme and terrifying fears many times in the past, thinking my family members were out to punish me. But this time I was terrified of the cat, believing he was seeking revenge because I had not fed him on time, because I had pushed him aside. I found myself cowering under his angry gaze, watching his every move, until eventually I managed to lock him outside, too frightened to be alone with him in the house.

Spiders, too, were out for revenge. They lay in every quiet, dark corner, just waiting for night-time when I turned the light off. Then they attacked, hordes of them lunging viciously at me because I had killed their families. I crept round the room, spraying insecticide in corners, in the wardrobe, under the bookcase and bed, checking under the mattress, under the pillow and then under the doona. I was too afraid to lie down and close my eyes.

I took Serenace for two days and the symptoms began melting away. My head cleared, my aggression and libido scuttled into their respective corners, and my vision returned to normal. Peace at last. Now I could sleep and the following day could be spent productively instead of wasted on the couch.

Before the holiday period started I had decided that a good part of my break would be spent writing this book, and with my mood now apparently quite normal, I felt I could be very productive.

I ploughed in, rereading and editing what I had already done, and continuing on with new work, reading and typing day and night. Sleep varied between two and five hours each night. I was not tired as such, but I recognised the fact that I was over-taxing myself because there were periods in each day when I developed double vision and nausea.

After a few days I began to wonder about my mood. I felt so *normal*, even peaceful, and my work was flowing so smoothly, that I decided I could not possibly be high. I completely ignored the fact that I had taken Valium two nights previously to stop the mental activity so that I could sleep.

I reflected on the week with more care as I reached its end. I realised that in fact my confidence, irritability, and mental activity were higher than normal, and that for at least a few of those nights I'd forgotten my evening medication, probably because I hadn't been eating regular meals, and medication is taken with meals.

I decided to take better care of myself but, because I was so productive, I also decided to leave my mood where it was and take no Serenace. I was 'on a roll' here and didn't want anything to spoil it. How wonderful it would be if we could capture our mood at just the level we want, or need, at a given point, and maintain it at that level.

1993

New Year's Eve found me sitting at my computer again. I was in a working mood, and not even invitations to New Year's parties could persuade me to move. For the next five days, apart from spending one day with a Greek woman-friend who was holidaying in Melbourne, I sifted through notes and journal entries, reading and typing as I went. My mind was churning over at a great rate, and I slept no more than four hours any night.

By the end of the five days I had completed my targeted quantity of work and was content to go no further for the moment. It was time now to take a break from the computer. I was suffering a lot of visual disturbance and a migraine threatened.

I decided that my energies needed to be channelled into something physical and over the next few days I tried working in the garden (which was again becoming an obsession), sewing, housework and moving furniture around. Just when I began to fear that I was again in the mood to spend, luck stepped in and saved me from myself. My mood slipped down a few notches and I was not the slightest bit interested in shopping.

At my next visit to Dr W., it was decided that if and when I next slipped into a high, I should take a larger dose of Serenace and for an extended period of time. He also instructed me that at the first signs of poor sleep, wanting to spend money, elevated libido or becoming obsessive, I was to ring him so that precautions could be taken before any damage was done. With this course of action planned, and having no credit facilities, no cash, and a mountain of debts to pay off, I felt confident that my spending days were indeed over.

The holidays were soon behind me and I returned to work, still in an elevated mood and eager to start working again. I sensed that 1993 was to be the major turning point in my illness, that again there would be a noticeable improvement. The year was to hold more highs than lows, with few of the fluctuations being severe or causing great problems in spite of one splurge when I spent over $1500 on prints, paintings, plants and other odds and ends. This was the first, and hopefully the last, occasion when my cheques would bounce – my usual credit facilities at banks and the supermarket had been temporarily suspended.

In February, tests by a cardiologist revealed that I had developed aberrant conduction in the intraventricular pathways. Mogens Schou, in *Lithium Treatment of Manic-Depressive Illness*, says that changes of the function or electrical activity of the heart are occasionally seen during Lithium treatment, but the presence of heart disease rarely prevents well-motivated Lithium treatment of manic-depressive illness. Whether or not Lithium was the cause of my problem remains unclear. Medication was prescribed for this condition and I was ordered to immediately stop smoking. This was very difficult and my anxiety level increased dramatically. I also became very aggressive when my mood was elevated, once flying into a terrible rage, smashing cups and attacking the kitchen bench and chopping board with a carving knife. I was frightened because I had very little control, and the mood lasted for quite some time. However, once again Serenace helped to control the situation, as it has on many occasions since then.

The severity and duration of my depressive moods seemed to have eased dramatically by this time, although during one episode my memory was exceedingly poor, and I became very confused about everyday things, such as suddenly thinking plastic $10 notes were in circulation, quite a long time before they came into existence. Also, I forgot how to manipulate the car's steering wheel when I was turning corners. I was very confused, about this and many other situations, unable to recall what had previously been done automatically. I completely forgot the names of people I worked with every day, and if I had to provide change, the client often had to prompt me or actually do it for me. But, as usual, I passed it off with a smile and comments such as 'Oh dear, I'm not quite awake yet' or 'I'm having one of *those* days'.

My mind began to turn constantly to old age which I, although only forty-eight, perceived as being just around the corner. I became anxious about my future state of health, thinking I would very soon be in need of 'care', and started to investigate retirement villages.

In May I was taken off Lithium and Tegretol, firstly because I had again developed Lithium toxicity, and secondly because I was now using cortisone cream daily to combat the severe and persistent allergic-type rashes over my scalp, face and body, caused by the Tegretol. Dr W. decided to try another anticonvulsant, Epilim. Over the next few months I showed a marked improvement but, unfortunately, the Epilim was causing my white blood count to drop to an unhealthy level and it, too, had to be discontinued. So it was back to Lithium, the old faithful, which I am still taking.

1994 and onwards

At the time of writing, my mood usually fluctuates between twenty per cent above and twenty per cent below normal (see page 67), with some periods of being in a mild mixed state. If I were a computerised being, I would say my default setting for mood is now generally twenty per cent below normal. Taking the variations into account, including the 'normal' days, I have come to find this level quite acceptable as I am able, by focusing on work, other people, and other interests, to function capably in my busy, stressful administrative position, and even to pursue studies. At times my energy levels are low, of course, but I rest whenever I need to. 'Listening' to one's body and tending to its requirements are essential (see chapter 13).

Why on earth am I studying, when maintaining a job is more than many can manage? Well, thanks to this illness, I have become even more acutely aware of the fact that we all experience turbulent periods in our lives, and many struggle without support. I hope that my storehouse of life experience and newly acquired Diploma of Psychology and Diploma of Professional Counselling, as well as voluntary helping and counselling work of the past twelve months, will provide me with the opportunity to help and support others in a practical way. I may even be able to pursue further studies in the area of psychology.

It would be easy to sit back and let my mood wash over me at times (a natural tendency with melancholia), but I recognise that if I did, I would sink further into introspection and isolation, achieving nothing. I want to experience life, not isolation. I have a lot to offer, and in fact, by studying and/or working, I am actually protecting myself – as long as I keep things in proper perspective and 'listen' to the needs of my body, mind and soul.

> In her autobiography, *Blackberry Winter: My Earlier Years*, Margaret Mead talked of how, having been excluded from sorority life at college, she learnt what it meant both to exclude and to be excluded. It gave her empathy, she wrote, for those people who felt excluded and lonely.

> We may learn many things in our lives, but those things that are seared on the soul, the ones that have been most painful for us, provide us with a source of sensitivity and a greater sense of others' fragility. They allow us to understand and to enter another person's experience without intruding, because we feel their pain with them. (*The Self Alone*, Angela Rossmanith).

> In the words of R. Tagore, quoted in *Noon to Nightfall* by M. d'Apice:

'There is rain in your soul, my friend, and I have no umbrella. But let me walk beside you for a while.'

To experience suffering of any kind is to know the anguish other people can experience, and if this is the only thing to be learned from deep tormenting illness, then it is not a total waste of that suffering. To be able to recognise the rain in someone's soul, to be unable to offer the solution, yet still to be prepared to walk alongside for a while, is a sign of great sensitivity and compassion. Too few of us take the time to observe or contemplate the fragility of the deepest hidden recesses of the hearts and souls around us that need so much nourishment. Too many of us are engrossed in working at such a frantic pace simply for the material things in life that our eyes are not open to the real treasures of life that are so enriching – our fellow humans, why they are the way they are, writers' use of very ordinary words to touch our hearts, the subtle scent of a delicate rose glistening velvety in the early morning dew.

I do not know what the future has in store for me, yet I am content that the illness has finally stabilised at an acceptable level. I can continue to be productive, and my outlook is one of confidence. I have always considered myself to be empathic, but now the words of Tagore are etched forever in my heart and on my soul. I wish to live and breathe his words, so my past eight years have definitely not been a total waste of time. I am also fortunate that I have the ambition to strive and achieve (sometimes to my detriment) and, since the onset of my illness, have been forced to look into the very depths of my nature and learn to modify many aspects of that nature in order to survive. This has also been to my advantage.

Dr Anthony Clare says:

'... individuals with manic-depression frequently have a compensatory energy, drive and ambition ... associated with high social class and achievement and ... in one study of various categories of mood disorder, the epidemiologist Christopher Bagley found members of the professional and managerial classes were significantly over-represented.

Energy, drive and ambition cannot be experienced until either one is completely well again, or the illness is stabilised at an acceptable level. Now that the latter is the case with me, I am sure that whatever natural talents God has given me, together with what He has enabled me to learn from my illness, will ensure that I go on to pursue whatever goals I set for myself, and to continue learning about myself and about others.

Faith to believe
when within and without
There's nameless fear
in a world of doubt ...

9 Treatment and m
of mood diso

Anxiety and panic disorders

If you suffer from mild anxiety, the best cure is
are aware that something specific, such as your job or your relationship,
is responsible for your anxiety, then do all in your power to deal with the
situation, obtaining help if necessary.

Minor tranquillisers and anti-anxiety drugs

If you are in an anxiety state and can find no cause, you should consult
your doctor. Anti-anxiety drugs, or minor tranquillisers, will probably be
prescribed initially. These tranquillisers, originally developed to replace
barbiturates, provide relief from the anxiety and also from the
accompanying insomnia. Unfortunately, these drugs tend to be over-
prescribed and, because of the side effects and withdrawal symptoms, you
should be wary of taking them over a long period.

Side effects and dependence: Some people take minor tranquillisers
only at night to promote a good night's sleep, which then helps them to
get through the following day. Others take them throughout the day, and
perhaps also at night, and will often feel quite drowsy. For many, it is a
welcome relief to be slowed down this way, to have the edge taken off
their anxiety symptoms. Others find it difficult to work in this state.

Other side effects include lack of co-ordination, poor concentration,
impaired memory, palpitations, blurred vision, and fatigue.

In Australia today, prescriptions for minor tranquillisers account for
approximately five per cent of all Pharmaceutical Benefits Scheme

prescriptions. Approximately one third of the population have used minor tranquillisers at some time, and an estimated five to seven per cent of people take these drugs on a continuing daily basis. Women are prescribed twice as many as men, and people in the over-65 age group receive the most scripts. This is a worrying situation.

People taking them regularly over a long period (longer than two to three months) can become very dependent on them. Apart from the psychological difficulty of letting go, there is also a physical reaction when they are withdrawn, even when no more than a normal prescribed dose is being taken. For this reason, it is important to withdraw them slowly. A treating doctor or psychiatrist, a member of Tranquilliser Recovery and New Existence Inc (TRANX), a community health worker or alcohol and drug addiction worker will advise on the best way to do this, depending on the particular drug being used. Sometimes, for example, there is a need to reduce by half a tablet each week, then by a quarter and so on. If it is not done this way, symptoms such as shakiness, jitteriness, palpitations, sweating, headaches, urinary symptoms such as frequency and burning, hypersensitivity to light, noise, touch and smell, sleeping difficulties, and increased levels of anxiety will appear, and the temptation arises to again reach for those little pills. However, these symptoms will be minimised, and eventually will disappear, if a very slow rate of reduction under careful and constant supervision is maintained.

Not all people experience withdrawal symptoms, and certainly not all experience *all* of the above. Obviously, limited or short-term use of minor tranquillisers can be both helpful and necessary in the treatment of anxiety, and many people, under the guidance and supervision of their doctor, use these drugs without any problems at all. It is their long-term continuous use by uninformed patients that promotes dependence and its often disastrous consequences.

It should also be noted that some people experience withdrawal symptoms while still taking their normal dose because their bodies have become accustomed to the drug and require more to have the same effect. This is not always made clear to the patient when drugs are being prescribed. You should always ensure that you are made fully aware of the consequences and side effects of any prescribed medication. Do not be afraid to ask questions. Many doctors over-prescribe to the detriment of their patients.

A major problem can also arise when alcohol is combined with tranquillisers. The two interact with the body in much the same way as barbiturates, and can stay in the bloodstream for as long as eight days. The combination can lead to over-sedation and even coma in initial doses. Long-term problems in this area are a separate issue. Some very prominent people, such as former US First Lady Betty Ford, entertainers Liza Minelli and Elizabeth Taylor, and film-maker Barbara Gordon, have publicly acknowledged their problems with prescription drugs and alcohol in an effort to help others acknowledge and seek help for their drug and alcohol related problems. So alcohol and tranquillisers should never be mixed.

After taking tranquillisers for many months, even years, people find that withdrawal symptoms take many, many weeks, even months, to disappear. If all this sounds very off-putting remember, firstly, that an experienced professional will be able to guide you through withdrawal correctly and, secondly, if you decide that drugs are not for you no matter what, you can discuss with that person the other avenues available to you. Of course, there are those whose anxiety and depression are such that, although they do not want to take tranquillisers, they find there is no alternative in the short term to enable them to carry on with their daily lives. It should be borne in mind, however, that these tranquillisers will not rid a person of anxiety the way antibiotics rid the body of an infection. They provide only temporary relief.

How do you know if you have become dependent on tranquillisers? If any of the following danger signs apply to you, you may be dependent on your pills:

- You have been taking tranquillisers or sleeping pills for six months or longer, continuously.
- Your doctor has increased your dose.
- You are taking doses larger than those recommended.
- You are getting extra pills from different doctors.
- You always make sure you have an adequate supply of pills and carry them on you 'just in case'.
- You have taken more than one brand of minor tranquilliser.
- You take one or two extra pills when you know you have to face a stressful situation.
- You are mixing your pills with alcohol or other drugs.
- The drug is interfering with your life in some way, causing difficulties in family relationships or social life.

- You have tried unsuccessfully to cut down your dose or to stop taking your pills altogether.

As a general rule, it is best if tranquillisers are used as a means of relieving the anxiety while you find other methods of dealing with it, much the way you might initially take a pain-killer to relieve a migraine while you find ways of dealing with the stress that you think has caused it.

If you think you have become dependent on your tranquillisers and are experiencing withdrawal difficulties, don't feel guilty and ashamed. Seek help immediately from a professional person you can trust, or from one of the organisations that exist to help people with drug dependencies. Never try to stop taking your tranquillisers without professional supervision – to do so could be dangerous.

Remember that minor tranquillisers act on the brain and central nervous system, which control all systems of the body and, in withdrawal, all parts of the body are affected. Your body has become accustomed to functioning with the drugs, and when you stop taking them, it goes 'haywire' for a short time. This is withdrawal. But you *will* recover, and your body and mind *will* return to normal functioning in time and with careful supervision and support.

As already noted, I have used tranquillisers from time to time, both at the onset of, and during, the more crippling episodes of my panic attacks. For a time I certainly was dependent on them. Obviously I would have preferred to cope without them, but even in retrospect, I know there were times when they were absolutely essential for my continued functioning. I qualify these comments by saying that being treated by my particular psychiatrist made drug-taking less objectionable. He, specialising in these drugs of addiction and preferring that I not take them at all, was always careful to acquaint me with the side effects and always carefully monitored my dosage and withdrawal. Nevertheless, it afforded me great satisfaction to be able, in the latter part of 1990, to discontinue Xanax and Valium, and to have been virtually free of them since.

Therapies and self-help

Professor Graham D. Burrows and Fiona K. Judd, in 'Panic and phobic disorders', suggest that supportive psychotherapy in which the patient takes an active role is essential, as many people suffering panic disorder or agoraphobia and panic attacks have severe interpersonal problems. They suggest that appropriate therapy consists of a combination of pharmacological and psychological treatments. Pharmacological agents used in the treatment of anxiety include tricyclic antidepressants, monoaminoxidase inhibitors, benzodiazepines, beta blockers and, more recently, the triazalo-benzodiazepine, alprazolam (Xanax), which has been shown to be rapidly effective in the treatment of panic attacks. Xanax has considerable advantages over the antidepressants, with far fewer side effects.

Once the attacks are controlled, anticipatory anxiety and phobic avoidance might resolve without specific intervention. A number of people will continue to experience severe forms of these conditions, and for these people pharmacological and psychological measures to control generalised anxiety, and behavioural psychotherapy for the treatment of phobic avoidance, will be necessary.

It would be wise to explore the various types of therapies and other methods of treatment that are available to help people with anxiety or drug dependence problems. Hypnotherapy, acupuncture, meditation, relaxation and yoga are just some that have proved beneficial adjuncts for some people. Consider, too, the various self-help methods such as those mentioned below, or you may wish to approach one of the organisations listed at the back of this book.

There are a number of methods described in books on library shelves to help overcome fears, phobias and general anxiety. I have tried most of them in an effort to cure my anxiety. Those I have found to be the most helpful, down-to-earth and practical are the step-by-step methods put forward by Dr Claire Weekes in her book *Self Help for Your Nerves,* the Morita therapy as described by psychotherapist Betty McLellan in her book *Overcoming Anxiety*, and the very comprehensive *Living with Anxiety* by Dr Bob Montgomery and Dr Laurel Morris, a book that deals not only with anxiety, phobias and agoraphobia, but also with obsessive-compulsive problems, post-traumatic stress disorder, and strengthening social, sexual and interpersonal skills.

Betty McLellan acknowledges the similarities between the Morita method and that of Dr Weekes, and all methods are based on facing and accepting the anxiety rather than fighting it, in much the same way the alcoholic attending Alcoholics Anonymous accepts the condition by saying 'I am an alcoholic'. The next step is focusing on practical action. From that moment, when you have stopped steeling yourself for daily battle, you will find the relief that comes with self-awareness and self-acceptance, and you can begin the journey back to good health.

However, when a person's anxiety is complicated by serious mental illness or chronic depression, these methods may not be so successful. Betty McLellan explains that this is because an important prerequisite for the success of the treatment is the anxiety-sufferer's commitment to the process, and those whose anxiety is complicated by any of the above conditions usually lack the kind of commitment required.

She recommends that those who suffer from any kind of psychotic illness should work (with a psychiatrist) towards the stabilising of the psychosis before attempting to commit themselves to the Morita process, and those suffering chronic depression are advised to try to work through their depression first with a psychotherapist or psychiatrist. Once these illnesses have been stabilised, it will be easier to find the dedication and patience required to work through the anxiety or agoraphobia with whatever method is chosen.

While some people will be able to work through a self-help method without assistance, many others will find it a long, arduous and lonely road to travel unless they are using it merely as an adjunct to the methods of treatment being adopted by their doctor or therapist. In any case, it is always advisable to keep your treating physician informed of any measures you decide to adopt outside his or her chosen methods. Success is likely to be achieved more rapidly and permanently if you both work together in an open and informed manner.

Wendy, who suffers from anxiety and manic-depression, has shown that she eventually found the required courage and commitment to work through her anxiety and panic attacks:

> I force myself to go for a swim when I feel afraid of water. I make myself go into the supermarket when I know I can't cope. When I don't come out with what I need, I tell myself it was a great effort to try when the [brain] chemicals are out of kilter.

She tells herself:

- No one can see what you are thinking.
- Just go slowly but make a start.
- You do have value – you're a mother, grandmother, daughter, friend, worker.
- This is just another of life's challenges.

Wendy's first two statements regarding swimming and going into the supermarket whilst being so afraid follow the advice of the self-help programs mentioned above, in that Wendy has learned to accept and face her fears. It is difficult at first, but gradually becomes easier.

Some minor tranquillisers and anti-anxiety drugs are listed in the table below.

Generic name	Australian trade name
alprazolam	Xanax
cobazam	Frisium
chlordiazepoxide	Librium
chlorazepate	Tranxene
diazepam	Antenex, Ducene, ProPam, Valium
fluzapam	Dalmane
lorazepam	Ativan
oxazepam	Serepax

Phobias

Apart from the initial use of tranquillisers to relieve the anxiety suffered by people with a severe phobia, there are other forms of professional treatment available, namely the desensitisation method and the flooding method.

Desensitisation method

Those with a severe phobia will more than likely be offered this treatment method. It takes longer to work than the flooding method but is less traumatic. It involves gradual exposure to the object of your fear, starting with a non-threatening situation where the object or situation is a safe distance from you, and progressing gradually to a stage where you are able to confront the most distressing situation and deal with it positively. You might first be asked to make a list of situations that are causing you distress, starting with the least frightening and finishing with the one that causes you the most anxiety. If you are afraid of spiders, for example, the least frightening exposure might be a spider sitting in its web on the back fence. Next on the list might be that same spider spinning a web on an overhanging branch near the pathway. Next could be the spider clinging to the wall by the back door, and the final situation on your list may be the spider suddenly appearing on the table in front of you. Once you have compiled your list, you are taught deep muscular relaxation before being asked to face the object of your fear.

You would then be asked to visualise in your mind the spider on the back fence. When you start to feel anxiety, you stop and practise relaxation. Then you again visualise the spider in the web, alternating visualisation and relaxation until the spider no longer causes you any distress. You then proceed through the list of distressing situations, dealing with each in the same manner.

The next step would be to go through similar processes using pictures or slides, and then, when you are comfortable looking at pictures, you would be exposed to spiders in real life, first with another person, then by yourself, always starting with the least threatening and working your way through to the most discomforting, until you are able to face any situation without being overcome by fear.

Flooding method

With this method, the person is virtually 'thrown in at the deep end'. Instead of being exposed gradually to their fear, they are asked to confront it head-on and then work through the distress. This was the method used effectively, without any tranquillisers, to cure my traffic phobia some twelve years ago following my motor vehicle accident. It is a highly stressful way of dealing with the phobia, but is often a better choice of therapy, as it was in my case.

As with desensitisation, the steps to be taken in the flooding method can also be first carried out in the mind, and I always found this quite helpful before each daily trip in the car. I visualised myself sitting behind the wheel of the car whilst parked outside the house, watching the traffic passing by. Then I visualised myself driving around the block, then the short distance to work, and later on a 20-minute drive from home, picturing all the stops at traffic lights along the way, changing lanes, passing other traffic and so on, and finally I imagined I was driving on the dreaded freeway, my biggest fear. But there was not much time for visualisation because, right from the word go, my doctor set specific weekly targets for me out on the road in all the situations I found the most fearful, and I had no choice but to work through my fears as I drove. It was frightening and exhausting, but it did work.

Afraid of flying?

As many as twenty per cent of our population are afraid of flying. Some are apprehensive about heights, others dislike being in enclosed spaces, while many have concerns about the safety of flying. For these people, there is a very good book available, written by Captain Robert Miles, a retired commercial airline pilot with more than twenty-seven years in the air, called *Conquer Fear of Flying* and illustrated by cartoonist WEG. Captain Miles wrote this book because he was concerned about the obvious distress of some passengers, and the book provides a wealth of information to dispel any fears people might have, as well as covering practical suggestions such as how to relax whilst in the air, what to wear for comfort, and so on.

Ansett Australia's Fear of Flying Program is also a highly effective means of conquering this fear. Five-week courses, consisting of a two and a half hour session per week, are held at the airports in Sydney, Melbourne, Brisbane, Adelaide and Perth. The program, which enjoys a ninety per cent success rate, is conducted by a psychologist assisted by Ansett pilots, flight attendants and engineering staff. It covers all aspects of flight, training of pilots, traffic control, maintenance and safety, and also includes sessions that focus on the nature and development of fear, with participants learning relaxation techniques and procedures to control their anxiety-provoking thinking.

Agoraphobia

As with a general anxiety state, the initial use of tranquillisers in the treatment of agoraphobia is helpful, but the sufferer must eventually seek help from a doctor, therapist, professional or support organisation, use one of the self-help methods available, or a combination of self-help and professional help.

An essential element in effecting a recovery is *a willingness to change*, to change one's behaviour and way of thinking, and to accept responsibility for one's own recovery. It is necessary to develop sufficient confidence to set and pursue goals, and to achieve chosen aims. This is difficult to do alone, but with professional help success is possible.

Dr Claire Weekes, in her book *Simple Effective Treatment of Agoraphobia* (1977), puts forward her very successful method of dealing with this crippling problem. It would be ideal if a therapist could be found who is prepared to follow this or a similar method, but Dr Weekes' book, based on treatment by 'remote direction', has proved to be highly successful. It follows on from her first two books *Self Help for Your Nerves* and *Peace from Nervous Suffering*. Her description of the symptoms and step-by-step treatment method are clear and easy to understand and, in themselves, bring relief to the sufferer In that she or he immediately has something to relate to, and a down-to-earth method to follow. She gives many examples of others' experiences, and talks of the setbacks that can be expected and how to overcome them and move forward again.

She acknowledges the need for tranquillising at times, but says that learning how to cope with panic is essential for a permanent cure because 'once a person has suffered from nervous illness, memory, in an unguarded moment, can bring a return of panic in many different ways, places'.

Sufferers of anxiety and agoraphobia will often be advised to 'keep occupied' and, if they have a job, will be encouraged to keep working. In itself this is good advice because they will have their work colleagues, job responsibilities and social contacts to provide a distraction from the fear and to help keep life in some sort of perspective. However, it must also be remembered that although the agoraphobic person wants more than anything else to be busy and to be out in the world with other people, until they can learn with help to face their symptoms and not fear them, they will find it impossible to venture beyond their particular confining boundaries.

So the well-meant advice of keeping occupied will add to the anguish, as the individual is yet again made to realise that others do not understand his or her plight. Again, there will be self-doubt, and further eroding of self-esteem. There may be despair of ever being well again, and feelings of being forced to make some attempt to overcome the fear and to achieve some control. However, the state of mind at this time would cause great tension, and that very tension could possibly be the downfall of any attempts to move successfully beyond the security of regular boundaries. The person may venture out and go part of the way to a destination, only to be turned back by panic symptoms. The failure to achieve would cause more humiliation and despair, more hopelessness, and further withdrawal.

Unfortunately, by burying ourselves behind our secure boundaries, by not facing our fears and working our way through them, we are only prolonging the agony. We may feel less threatened, less fearful, but this is only temporary. Eventually the prospect of another terrifying situation will arise, and will have to make the decision to either face it and deal with it, or make some excuse to avoid it and remain locked in our world of fear, unable to enjoy the normal pleasures of life.

For those who really wish to understand agoraphobia and its associated panic attacks, and would like to help the sufferer, Bev Aisbett has some suggestions to make in *Living With IT – A Survivor's Guide to Panic Attacks* (Angus & Robertson, Sydney, 1994):

1. Listen. Panic People need to let it out. Often. Panic People need to talk it through. Often.
2. Encourage. Recognising that the Panic Person is trying will spur them on. Encourage them to keep going, but never bully them or become impatient. They are doing their best. They need your support.
3. Be the voice of reason. If the Panic Person is feeling chaotic, step in and guide them back to a point of focus. Encourage them to *think* rather than let their feelings run away them. Reason it out together.
4. Understand that this is very real to the Panic Person. There may be very severe physical symptoms.
5. Avoid surprises. The Panic Person needs to pace him/herself. They may need to plan ahead, so they can deal with each new situation.
6. Acknowledge each achievement. However small it may seem, to the Panic Person completing a new task may have meant climbing a mountain. Remind them, too, of their progress. They may forget at times.
7. Try to be patient. This is hard, but getting angry or showing frustration will only make the Panic Person feel guilty. It takes time and effort to change, and remember, you are well; you have more reserves to call on.
8. Become informed. It is a great help if you know about the strategies that will help the person through to recovery. You can then work with them to achieve their goal and return *both* your lives to normal.

(Reprinted with the permission of HarperCollins Publishers.)

It would appear that agoraphobic people tend by nature to be zealous, determined and sensitive people who set extremely high standards for themselves and who do not like falling short of their high expectations. So, by their very nature they are prone to fear, anxiety and tension, and have the fighting spirit necessary to overcome obstacles. But it is this same fighting spirit that now causes them so many problems because, to be free of fear and tension, they must stop fighting and adopt a relaxed attitude. To be phobic is to fight what is feared, and agoraphobic people do not understand that their permanent state of tension and anxiety is increasing the symptoms of fear, creating a vicious circle that is very difficult to break. Tranquillisers help initially, but eventually the agoraphobe must seek help to face his or her fears and work through them.

Manic-depressive illness

For some people, their first experience with mental health professionals occurs during an acute manic episode when hospitalisation is necessary. But for those who suffer depression initially, the illness will have crept up much more slowly, and they will probably approach their general practitioner because of symptoms such as sleep disturbance, fatigue and diminished sexual drive.

Once the general practitioner has recognised your symptoms he or she may prescribe medication immediately, or may refer you to a psychiatrist. The next step is to find a good psychiatrist with whom you feel comfortable, and one you feel confident will not over-prescribe drugs. Your general practitioner will no doubt have someone in mind, but you should feel free to ask for a referral to more than one psychiatrist. Visit one, and then another if necessary for a 'second opinion' and to make a comparison. If you do not feel happy or comfortable with either, ask to see a third. Ask questions of them all. If you are still not happy, keep searching, keep asking. You may have made your initial contact with mental health professionals through your local Community Health Centre. It may also be helpful at this stage to find a support group in your local area where others will be able to recommend professional people with whom they have dealt. One area where the respondents to my questionnaire are in strong agreement is, do not continue with a psychiatrist with whom you are not happy or with whom you do not feel comfortable for any reason.

I have often found it necessary to discuss with my psychiatrist my deepest and most intimate thoughts which I never have revealed, and never will again reveal, to another living being. Had I not been able to do this, I would have been so heavily burdened with guilt and self-loathing that I might have extinguished the flickering flame of life long ago. I know that I would never have been able to unburden myself to that extent with anyone other than a medically qualified doctor who had long been exposed to mental illness with all its quirks and manifestations. He was the one person who had seen in others what I was experiencing and could offer medical knowledge, understanding, comfort and support. No matter how hard anyone else tried, they could never look after me as a whole person, mentally and physically, as he did.

So, trust was the most important ingredient in the relationship – my ability to feel totally at ease with my doctor. His professional manner, his certainty with diagnosis, and his ever-caring manner, all instilled great confidence in me. Of course, there were times when I questioned and doubted him, even rejected his advice or treatment, but at all times I felt at ease to lay my cards on the table.

A good doctor–patient relationship takes time to build, and is not always easy for either party, but from the patient's point of view, it is imperative that a good rapport be established.

Professor Patrick D. McGorry in *The Concept of Recovery and Secondary Prevention in Psychotic Disorders* says that

> the value of psychotherapeutic relationships in all phases of psychotic illness cannot be underestimated. During the florid phase the patient is often difficult to contact, yet is in dire need of such contact, as well as support and understanding. During recovery and beyond, the establishment of a supportive psychotherapeutic relationship whose continuity is assured is essential in enabling the person to cope with and indeed survive the whole experience of the disorder. Within the context of such a relationship it is possible to help the person to focus upon the tasks relevant to their particular situation and phase of illness, and to help them to adapt and integrate without despair or 'engulfment' in the chronic patient role.

Quite obviously, then, there is a lot to be gained from a comfortable, harmonious doctor–patient relationship. Another important and practical way to ensure that you receive the best possible treatment is, between doctors' visits, to keep notes of all the problems you encounter, and any questions that you need answered. Do not rely on your memory, which is usually poor due to the illness itself and also the medication. Your doctor must know what is happening to you at all times if he or she is to properly treat you. Keeping a graph is also most helpful in this regard (see page 67).

When we initially consult a psychiatrist, the question of stigma crosses our minds, and we may discuss the matter with only our closest relatives and perhaps one or two close friends. Many people I have encountered are very wary of the psychiatric profession, ridiculing it, labelling the psychiatrists as drug-pushers. For the most part, these people know little or nothing of the profession, or the patients and illnesses it deals with. They are naturally frightened, even repulsed, by mental illness, often seeing the afflicted people as dangerous or sub-human. I have, for the most part, been criticised for seeing a psychiatrist and for drug-taking, but these people did not have sufficient knowledge about the nature of my illness and the required treatment. Unfortunately, they were often not prepared to listen or believe. I and many of the people who responded to my questionnaire are no longer bothered unduly by stigma, looking instead to public education to promote wider understanding.

Once you are seeing a psychiatrist, the mainstay of treatment will be medication. Some medications are used only for mania, some for depression, and others treat both. Some are used for long-term maintenance, some for short-term acute episodes. Each patient is treated according to his or her own needs and circumstances at a given time, and treatment might include medication alone, medication with psychotherapy, or less frequently, when the person has been stable for quite a long time, therapy alone.

Professor McGorry also points to the patient's own strengths and positive attributes as being vital elements in recovery. These would include the less tangible yet potentially healing qualities such as courage, perseverance, resourcefulness, humour, spirituality and creative skills as well as other more practical skills which have been used to successfully manage a previous crisis. He says that, ideally, the role of the patient should be as active as possible and indeed it is probably essential to the recovery process that patients play an active role in relation to their disorder and to the therapeutic interventions on offer. However, each person must be allowed to discover at their own pace a way of coming to terms with the new reality that they have developed a psychotic illness, a task which he acknowledges to be extremely difficult, one that would tax the strongest ego, requiring a great deal of assistance and forbearance while it is being negotiated.

Antidepressants

Tricyclic antidepressants: For those whose illness commences with a depressive episode, the first choice of medication is usually an antidepressant, with tricyclic antidepressants being the most commonly used. They are so named because there are three rings in their molecular structure. It appears that these drugs increase the effective quantity of monoamine neurotransmitters in the brain. They do not cure the depression, but control it, keeping the symptoms in check until the illness lifts of its own accord. For some unknown reason, although the side effects are noticeable immediately, the beneficial results do not become apparent for some weeks. It varies from person to person, but is usually within the range of three to six weeks.

Apart from a dry mouth, the side effects also vary from person to person, but are usually dry mouth, blurred vision, drowsiness, constipation, tremor, and changes in blood pressure that can lead to fainting on getting up too fast. Weight gain can also be a problem, partly perhaps because the medication has an effect on the metabolism, but also due to the fact that the depressed person often has an increased appetite for carbohydrates and sweet foods.

There are many of these antidepressants, with more coming onto the market all the time, but the table below names some of the well-known ones.

Generic name	Australian trade name
amitryptiline	Amitrip, Mutabon, Laroxyl, Tryptanol, Endep
clomipramine	Anafranil
desipramine	Pertofran
dothiepin	Prothiaden
doxepin	Deptran, Quitaxon, Sinequan
imipramine	Imiprin, Tofranil
nortryptiline	Nortab, Nortrip, Allegron
trimipramine	Surmontil

Other types of antidepressant drugs, known as monoamine oxidase inhibitors (MAOIs), are also available but to date have not been so widely used because of strict dietary restrictions are necessary because the MAOIs can interact dangerously with other substances in your system, producing a sudden and severe rise in blood pressure that causes severe headache. A stroke, or even death, can occur, although this is very rare indeed. Foods to be avoided are those containing tyramine, among them being matured cheeses and yeast extracts. There are a number of other banned foods, but most usually do not feature in a regular diet as cheese does. There are certain non-prescription medications that must also be avoided. It is unlikely, however, that a doctor would prescribe these MAOIs without providing a list of the banned foods and medications.

As patients, however, it is in our own interests always to ask questions of our doctor and pharmacist to make sure that we are not taking medications that interact dangerously, and to find out what restrictions are placed on us with each new medication that is prescribed for us.

Some MAOIs are given below.

Generic name	Australian trade name
iproniazid	Marsilid
isocarboxazid	Marplan
phenelzine	Nardil
tranylcypromine	Parnate

Of course, there are always new drugs coming onto the market, and among the recent successful ones that have very few, if any, side effects, is fluoxetine (Prozac 20). Prozac 20 is a highly selective inhibitor of serotonin uptake. Although all the tricyclic antidepressants inhibit the uptake of serotonin, they are not selective for this neurotransmitter. Similarly, the monoamine oxidase inhibitors inhibit the metabolism of other neurotransmitters in addition to serotonin. An important recent advance in the treatment of depression has been the development of highly selective inhibitors of serotonin uptake.

The major advantages of Prozac 20 are its lack of anticholinergic adverse effects such as dry mouth, blurred vision and constipation, and its relative safety in overdose. It can, however, produce nausea, insomnia, anxiety and headaches in some people.

Paroxetine (Aropax 20) is another new antidepressant. There is some evidence that it may be of therapeutic value in those who have failed to respond to standard therapy and it can improve associated symptoms of anxiety. Side effects are considered to be generally mild in nature and do not affect one's lifestyle.

Another new antidepressant is Aurorix. The chemical structure of Aurorix is unrelated to any other antidepressant, selectively inhibiting monoamine oxidase A, preventing the breakdown of serotonin, noradrenaline and dopamine, reduced levels of which have been linked to depression. Aurorix also causes few side effects, no weight gain even in long-term therapy, and does not cause dangerous interactions with food and other drugs.

Zoloft is the other new antidepressant that causes few, if any side effects, and to date has proved to work efficiently.

Always check with your doctor or pharmacist about the correct way to take your medication. Some medicines must be taken with food, others will be rendered useless if taken with drinks that contain tannin, such as tea, coffee or cola, while the tranquillising effect of some drugs may be neutralised or regulated by the caffeine in these drinks. In fact, Dr Andrew Campbell, Director of Clinical Services at Rozelle Hospital, told a Sydney mental health services conference that doctors should be warning patients against having these drinks within an hour of taking many common antipsychotic and antidepressant drugs. He also emphasised the fact that the interaction only occurred when the drugs were taken orally, not when injected.

Lithium: Lithium Carbonate is a simple salt found in rocks and water and, as with many medicines, no one really knows how it works. Its benefits for manic patients were discovered quite accidentally in 1949 by a Melbourne psychiatrist, Dr John Cade. Prior to this time there was no effective treatment for those manic patients who had to be physically restrained, and had to suffer their disabling manic episodes with only relatively ineffective and dangerous sedatives available to them. Seriously depressed persons had been receiving some relief since the 1930s when electroconvulsive therapy was introduced, but still nothing could be done to prevent recurrence of bipolar mood disorder until the advent of Lithium as a treatment.

There is only a small gap between the dose of the salt that is effective and the dose that is toxic, so it took quite some time for its use to be universally accepted. However, it is now considered to be the drug of choice in mania, and when used preventively, reduces the possibility of future episodes of mania and depression. Lithium keeps the illness under control rather than curing it, and if a patient stops taking her or his Lithium, episodes of the illness are likely to reappear as frequently and severely as before. About 1800 years ago, Greek physicians were treating manic patients by having them 'take' the waters of certain springs that still exist today and are known to contain Lithium.

People taking Lithium must have their serum lithium levels checked regularly. Blood samples are taken once a week during the first weeks, then at longer intervals according to the doctor's instructions. Lithium dosage varies from one person to another, and is based on the concentration in the blood serum and the patient's response to treatment. Lithium works only if it is in a sufficient concentration in the system, but serum levels must not be allowed to jump into the toxic range. The right level is called the 'therapeutic range', and it may take anything from two to eight tablets per day to reach this level.

Because of its effect on the kidneys, Lithium can produce excessive secretion of urine. This will make a person thirsty, and it is important to quench the thirst whilst taking Lithium, especially in hot weather, to avoid the risk of dehydration, which causes the blood level of lithium to rise. However, it would be wise to avoid high-calorie drinks such as cordial, milk or soft drinks which may quickly result in unwanted weight gain. It is also important to maintain salt intake at a normal level, so 'no salt' diets should be avoided. Diuretics, which affect the excretion of lithium by the kidneys, are also to be avoided unless your doctor has prescribed them and, if necessary, adjusted the Lithium dosage.

Increased thirst and urination, loss of appetite initially, fine tremor in the fingers and hands, weight gain and short-term memory loss are the most commonly reported side effects. However, should the thirst and urination become excessive, or the tremor very pronounced, or should you develop vomiting, severe diarrhoea, lack of co-ordination, slurred speech, confusion, or severe drowsiness, then you should immediately cease taking the Lithium, drink as much fluid as you can, and contact your doctor or go to a hospital. These are warning signs of impending toxicity.

In a small proportion of people, long-term Lithium treatment will lead to hypofunction of the thyroid gland. This is a risk that has to be accepted with long-term treatment, and the hypothyroidism that follows can be readily treated with thyroid extract.

Other medications: What of those bipolar sufferers, including some in the categories of rapid cycling and mixed state, who are treatment-resistant, who find the Lithium ineffective or cannot tolerate the side effects? Approximately thirty-three per cent of patients either cannot tolerate the side effects or do not show a satisfactory improvement with Lithium.

The drugs most commonly used in these cases are the anticonvulsant medications carbamazepine (Tegretol) and sodium valproate (Epilim) with carbamazepine being considered to be as efficient as Lithium. Phillip Mitchell, Professor of Psychiatry at Prince Henry Hospital Sydney, in *Current Therapeutics*, February 1992, advised:

> Initial interest in the use of anticonvulsants in mood disorders followed reports of the efficacy of carbamazepine for depression and anxiety in epilepsy. Open trials in Japan in the early 1970s by Okuma et al. suggested that carbamazepine possessed both antimanic and prophylactic properties for bipolar disorder ... About 80% respond either fully or partially to carbamazepine, with a delay action of about 7 to 14 days. Carbamazepine is often *added* to Lithium after a failure to respond to that medication, though it should be noted that side-effects are more common when the drugs are used in combination.

In talking about sodium valproate, Professor Mitchell says:

> A recent large open prospective study of lithium-resistant bipolar patients has indicated that sodium valproate is an effective prophylactic agent for this condition. That study suggested that sodium valproate was particularly effective in those with rapid-cycling bipolar disorder and in those with 'mixed states'.

Clonazepam (Rivotril), which is a benzodiazepine (Valium-type drug), has also proved beneficial, used mainly as an adjunct to Lithium, and of particular use in the treatment of acutely manic patients.

These drugs have been shown to be more effective against mania than against depression, bringing acute manic episodes under control within one to two weeks, which is comparable to Lithium.

For those who do not show sufficient response to either Lithium or anticonvulsants, a combination of both often proves beneficial.

The difficulty with this illness is that, although mania and depression present with quite different sets of symptoms, they are not two separate illnesses. They are merely two different features of the one illness, and must be addressed simultaneously if treatment is to be effective.

The side effects of Tegretol can be drowsiness, dizziness, ringing in the ears, increased sensitivity to sound, blurred or double vision, dry mouth, nausea, and diarrhoea or constipation, but these often disappear in time. Irritating skin rash can also be a problem, probably more so in those prone to allergies or asthma, and should also be mentioned to your doctor should it arise.

The side effects of Epilim, which may also resolve in time, tend to be nausea, stomach upset and diarrhoea, increased appetite and weight gain.

Clonazepam can produce drowsiness, lack of co-ordination, poor concentration, impaired memory, dizziness, loss of balance and blurred or double vision, nausea or dry mouth.

Most of the above symptoms do not occur, of course, and those that do occur vary from person to person and are usually quite mild.

The last group of medications that should be mentioned are those used in acute mania or psychotic depression, the antipsychotic (neuroleptic) drugs such as haloperidol (Serenace) or chlorpromazine (Largactil), which are used at times to reduce the symptoms quickly, or to ensure the person's safety. However these drugs are not suitable for long-term maintenance.

Dr Jonathan Upfal, in *The Australian Drug Guide*, advises that they calm the terror of psychosis, loosen the grip of delusory ideas, banish voice hallucinations, restore coherence to the thoughts and help re-establish emotional contact with others. Haloperidol is less sedating and has fewer 'drying' side effects than other major tranquillisers, but is more likely to cause some mild side effects such as abnormal movement and posture reactions such as 'restless legs', an inner compulsion to move continually, a general stiffness of posture, lack of expression, slowed movement and muscle tremor. These and other mild symptoms such as light-headedness, dizziness, drowsiness, mental dullness or blurred vision usually disappear during treatment, but the treating doctor should be advised if symptoms become troublesome or persistent. Also, a protective sunscreen lotion should be used on exposed skin to prevent a rash resembling sunburn, which sometimes occurs.

Another new antipsychotic drug now on the market is remoxipride hydrochloride (Roxiam), which causes side effects that are mild and transient and include drowsiness, tiredness, insomnia, concentration disturbances, dry mouth, headache, restlessness and anxiety.

Treatment resistance: When, after a reasonable period of time, a satisfactory response to a number of medications has not been forthcoming, the patient is considered to be treatment-resistant. The reasons for this are quite varied, but could include one or more of the following:

- side effects may reach intolerable levels
- the patient may fail to take the medication regularly or may discontinue medication
- there may be adverse drug interactions, alcohol or drug abuse
- there may be other medical conditions such as hypothyroidism or chronic fatigue syndrome which limit the effectiveness of medications
- there could simply be no response to the prescribed medication.

Response to any medication is highly individual, and a certain proportion of patients will fail to respond.

Electroconvulsive therapy (ECT)

For those patients with particular problems such as very severe depression not responding to medication, electroconvulsive therapy (ECT) (shock treatment) can be an alternative that produces remarkably quick and beneficial results. It has had its critics over the years, due to abuse and fear, but today's ECT is gentler than it used to be and is very effective. Certainly for those who are suicidal or suffering from delusions, it is often the treatment of choice, producing more rapid results than medication. Many people have testified to the benefits of ECT and are grateful that the choice was available to them.

Psychotherapies

Psychotherapy, basically, is talking with someone, removing symptoms by support and understanding, changing rigid behaviour patterns by a deeper exploration and understanding of yourself. It is a channel through which you can express your thoughts and feelings in a safe and controlled setting, and obtain feedback from the therapist, who has some objectivity and life experience. It provides a move from your usual restricting negative attitudes towards positive attitudes, and towards an acceptance of life, of yourself and your limitations.

There are a number of types of therapy and you should discuss these with your psychiatrist who will no doubt be giving you supportive therapy as a routine part of your treatment anyway. But if what you are receiving in the way of therapy from your psychiatrist seems lacking for your particular needs, then you should feel free to discuss the question of the other therapies that are available. It should be said here, however, that whilst a person in a mild to moderate depression ('grey depression') can be helped by therapy, it is useless for the person in a deep, or 'black', depression, who is unable to be reached by anyone – even a psychiatrist. Mild depression can usually be helped by human contact, whereas severe depression is aggravated by any intimacy.

Of the respondents to my questionnaire, eighty per cent said they received one or more types of therapy. Of those people, twenty-four per cent expressed dissatisfaction with the type of therapy received, fifty-two per cent found it generally very helpful, and twenty-four per cent found it extremely successful. A few whose parents or other family members had also suffered from the illness had obviously gained sufficient experience over time to feel no need for any therapy other than the supportive therapy of the treating psychiatrist.

Cognitive therapy: Cognitive therapy teaches patients to identify and change the way they think and improve overly pessimistic views of themselves and the world.

Interpersonal therapy: Interpersonal therapy focuses on current relationships and strategies for improving them. Its goal is to help patients develop more successful ways of relating to other people.

Behavioural therapy: Behavioural therapy emphasises self-monitoring, to make sure patients recognise and reward their own actions.

Family therapy: Family therapy provides a setting in which relatives can become more aware of each other's feelings and can see the impact of their own behaviour on other family members.

Some coping strategies for depression

The following strategies will work in milder forms of depression. They will not work in moderate to severe depression. Many sufferers, including myself, practise these basic principles with success.

- Make yourself get out of bed and, if possible, out of the house. The world has to be better outside your head.
- Break your time into manageable pieces, for example one day, half a day, one hour, depending on how you feel. Don't look at the clock and say 'Oh no! It's only eleven o'clock. How will I ever make it through

the day?' Think of something you can do for just half an hour or an hour so that you don't have to cope with the whole day.

- When you don't feel like doing something, *immediately do it without thinking about it,* for example when having a shower is too much to handle because you don't have the energy to wash and dry yourself, just *get out of the bed and into the shower* without thinking about it. It works!
- Cope with the problems of the *present* only, not the past or the future.
- As with time, break down tasks into manageable pieces. With housework, think to yourself, 'I'll just do the dishes.'
- When you are feeling down, get a piece of paper and a pen and write down how you feel. It can act as an outlet.
- Do something nice for someone else. It will make you feel better, even if it is just giving a rose or sending a card.
- Participate in a hobby, for example gardening, or just take your dog for a walk.
- Try to get a relaxation tape and *practise* – it can offer relief.
- Try to stop negative thoughts spiralling you downwards. When they enter your head, try to block them out with other thoughts or, better still, go and do something.
- Each night, try to think of a small thing you enjoy doing, and go to sleep knowing there is something to look forward to the next day.
- If you have a pool nearby, swimming or even just walking in the water is great – and good exercise as well.
- Try to be with other people – being alone can be a disaster.
- Remember when you are depressed to think, *'I've been through it before – I can do it again.'*

If you find these suggestions very hard to put into practice, don't worry; so have those before you. However, when tried, they can and do work, and should not be passed over as not worth the effort. There will be days, of course, when it is impossible to tackle even the most basic of these suggestions, those days when you must 'go with the flow', do what is best for you at that particular moment, even if it means spending the day in bed. What works one day may not work the next, and what works for one person may not work for another.

Most importantly, you should never feel that you are lazy or guilty if you are not able to tackle the daily tasks that you would normally be able to cope with. These guilt feelings only compound your distressing situation. We all go through very, very long stages, particularly following the onset of depression, of feeling incapable of even walking from the bed to the door. It is all too much of an effort, physically and mentally. Sometimes this stage lasts months at a time, sometimes years, on and off. So *please, please* do *not* feel guilty when you cannot do what you think you ought to be doing. This total depletion of energy, these guilt feelings, are all a natural part of the illness. You should allow yourself to be wrapped in cotton wool and nurtured, if that is what you need at the time. Usually it takes many years of illness to come to this conclusion. It did with me – and so if I can help *you* to accept your illness for what it is, and knock the guilt on the head, then I will be very happy.

General management

Each person must learn to recognise the symptoms that herald an impending mood swing, called 'prodromal symptoms' or early warning signs. This is important but often very difficult, because an illness that affects mood and thought processes, by its very nature, makes it exceedingly difficult for the person to know which are normal mood changes and valid feelings, and which are not. Discussion with the psychiatrist will help in this regard, and once the person is able to recognise an impending shift in mood he or she can immediately notify the psychiatrist who can make any necessary readjustment to the medication and, hopefully, prevent the looming episode or at least lessen its effects.

In this respect, a person should always be watchful if he or she decides to stop taking medication for any reason. This is quite a common occurrence, as many people, thinking they have been 'well' for some time, will decide to go off the drugs, testing their limitations. This can often, but not always, result in further episodes, as it has with me occasionally, and if the person is not acutely aware of the symptoms and on the lookout for them, may soon be back to where he or she originally was but with an even greater sense of hopelessness. The best advice here is that, if you do wish to stop taking your medication for any reason, you should discuss the matter with your doctor.

The effects of these illnesses vary from person to person. We each have individual needs and, as such, should avail ourselves of the various resources offered within the community to achieve a greater understanding of our illness and to make informed decisions about our preferred methods of treatment and management.

Many of the organisations at our disposal offer a library, videos and newsletters that keep us abreast of current mental-health issues, self-help and support groups for sufferers, carers and relatives, counselling (including telephone counselling services), seminars and workshops. Vocational retraining programs are also available to help people who want to return to the workforce.

Apart from offering information, these organisations and groups also provide an opportunity to share experiences, to learn from those who have already recovered, and to help others. In this way we no longer feel isolated, and are able to get things into proper perspective.

Just long enough for me to find
a little order in my life –
a little peace.

Vincent van Gogh

10 Hospitalisation

Vincent van Gogh understood the value of isolation from the world when he said he wanted to commit himself to an asylum, 'Just long enough for me to find a little order in my life – a little peace'.

The images that come to mind when psychiatric hospitals are mentioned can cause great fear, thanks to a few isolated stories sensationalised by the press, and the dramatic, sometimes horrifying, films produced by Hollywood. But these hospitals exist today for the same reason as any other hospital – to treat the sick. It is a safe environment where a team of professionals can diagnose, and provide medication and treatment whilst monitoring the patient's progress round the clock, which is not possible if the person is at home. The aim is to return the patient to family and community as quickly as possible.

Leonie Manns, of the Mental Health Co-ordinating Council, who was afflicted with manic-depressive illness, experienced a positive outcome to her suffering whilst hospitalised:

> I lie on the bed, legs curled up in an almost foetal position with my arms wrapped around my knees, just staring at the wall. The paint is peeling from the wall because the place is old and smells of ammonia and disinfectant. The bed is covered with the ubiquitous hospital bedspread. The whole place, even the occupants, is weighted down with that 'black hole' depression. I am in hospital again but this time I don't care as I am just too tired – actually I hope that they lock me up as I don't want to even try any more.

> I can't figure out why I keep ending up in hospital. One minute I am leading the most fantastic life. I have a great job (sometimes more than one), a nice flat with beautiful things around me and great friends and lovers. Life appears to be one long party. Then for no apparent reason things fall apart – I stop seeing my friends. I stay inside and I read and I eat and I feel that

blackness coming. Then I try to die – again. Then I'm here (or some other hospital) and it all starts again. This time though I am hoping it will stop because I don't want to be 'a good girl' any more – I just want to give up and let them lock me away.

I'm not asleep but I'm not awake either. I'm waiting. Then the doctor (one more in the long line) comes into the room. He sits down and starts to talk. I half listen and hear a few gobbledegook medico words but I take no notice until I hear him mutter something about '… under control … medication … feel better …' I sit up and ask him to start again. He tells me that I am suffering from a bipolar disorder that they think is caused by a chemical imbalance in the brain and that with correct treatment and medication this illness can be controlled.

I think that this sounds very feasible and begin my research into manic-depressive illness. Reading the literature is like reading my life story. At first I am angry. Why was this not found in other hospitals and by other doctors? Why? But this attitude was unproductive so I began to think more positively and immediately felt better, in fact I felt good because at last I knew what was wrong and that it wasn't my fault. I can't put my past back together but at least I feel that I now have a life. So I am 'living' with a mental illness.

The majority of people, even those with moderate to severe manic-depressive illness, do not require hospitalisation if treated in time with the correct medication, but there are times when a stay in hospital is either necessary or beneficial for the person's comfort or safety.

In depression, when movement, thought and speech are so slowed down that it becomes impossible to cope, and family tensions run high because the other members are so frustrated in their efforts to help, a period in hospital under the care of professional staff can provide a necessary respite for all concerned. And if suicidal thoughts have been present, as they often are in severe depression, the person is much safer in hospital being monitored twenty-four hours a day.

In a manic state, if a person cannot control his or her impulses, whether they be of a sexual nature, reckless spending or even violence, then hospitalisation becomes necessary to put a brake on the impulsive behaviour which might otherwise have a devastating effect on personal relationships, career and financial situation, and the family unit.

If a person is in the psychotic stage of mood disorder, then she or he will need the care and supervision that only skilled professionals can give, as may the person who has been living alone and whose physical as well as mental condition has deteriorated due to neglect.

Hospitalisation for the treatment of this illness still carries a stigma in some areas of the community. A person will have enough difficulty coming to terms with the fact of mental illness without having to face what is perceived as the 'shame' of being hospitalised for its treatment.

A number of private psychiatric hospitals now exist as well as private hospitals that have psychiatric wards. These wards are similar to other wards in the hospital: there are private rooms available with full facilities including attached bathroom, and there are no locked wards.

Hospitals these days offer programs that not only fill in the day constructively, but also maintain or improve functioning in all areas of day-to-day living. These programs generally include creative pursuits, group discussions, relaxation, stress management sessions, and social skills training, all of which are organised by nursing staff, occupational therapists and psychologists.

When I entered the foyer of my particular hospital in September 1989, there were no fears of what was to come. For a short time it would be a welcome sanctuary where I could, hopefully, break the vicious circle of trying to function, failing, trying again and failing, and becoming more and more anxious each time. It was 'time out' from work, and particularly from home, where tensions abounded and anxiety was rampant. It was an opportunity for me to recoup some strength and composure in safe and restful surroundings, whilst at the same time offering the family a respite from the tensions and disorder in their lives.

I found that being in hospital brought a great feeling of security. I was with people who suffered similar problems and staff who were used to dealing with those problems. Here I could just be myself without fear of anyone being judgmental, without losing the respect of those around me. I was in a place where I no longer had to worry about my inability to function properly in everyday life – I had only myself to think about. I did not even have the responsibility of remembering to take my medication. This hospital provided programs to aid in building, among other things, the patients' concentration, socialisation, living skills, self-esteem and stress management. The whole ward came together, with each person being actively involved in various parts of the daily program. There was a timetable on the wall of the lounge room, and we were each responsible for getting ourselves to the various activities on time.

However, during this particular stay, I refused to attend these programs. Having been involved in art and creative pursuits all my life, attending the creative classes meant going back to kindergarten standard, and I'd been used to Jane Fonda when I was high, so that doing gentle exercises on the floor or seated in a chair seemed a total waste of time. As for the discussion groups, or ward meetings as they were called, they required social interaction which I found too stressful at this stage.

I gave the staff a very difficult time, until they finally relented and left me to my own devices.

During my second stay in that hospital, however, which was only days after my initial discharge, the staff were more insistent, and because I was high and therefore in a more convivial frame of mind I agreed to their requests to join in all the activities except the creative classes, but as the days passed, I even took pleasure in the sense of achievement of other patients as they acquired new skills in the creative classes. The men, in particular, were often very eager to talk of their successes with craft work they had not previously been exposed to.

The one group session I found impossible to cope with was the relaxation session with the psychologist. Those of us who were going to join in would turn up with our pillows and make ourselves comfortable on his office floor. Some patients found it beneficial and actually reached the stage of dozing off, but my inner motor was too highly revved. Even when I had been brought out of my high, these sessions were difficult.

With the various activities going on, plus daily supervised trips out into the community for those who were able and interested, there was not a lot of time left to be idle, but I always found time to be alone in the garden which I had come to love so much, usually reading or writing. Most of the patients were in private rooms with their own TV so there was never a huge congregation in the lounge room in the evenings, but a few could always be found, often appearing to be in the throes of depression, just sitting, rarely talking.

After some days had passed, and I was no longer considered too great a risk, I was allowed out for afternoon walks and, of course, I had to pass by the local shops – in particular an antique shop that captured my attention immediately. Had I been in possession of much money or credit cards, there is no doubt that I would have been spending. As it was, the ten dollars I did have was spent on a pretty fruit bowl from the antique shop, which I filled with fruit and kept near my bed. It somehow took the edge off the craving to spend and gave me a sense of satisfaction.

But my afternoon excursions were always monitored by the ever-watchful staff who carefully checked me before I set out, and again on my return. I was allowed only a limited amount of time, and of course I had only very limited funds, and they knew when that had been spent, so there was never any danger of getting myself into any further trouble.

So, yet again, it was confirmed in my mind that hospitals are places that restore us to good health, where we can rest and recuperate before getting on with life again. Most, but certainly not all, of the respondents to my questionnaire stated that a stay in hospital had, at times, been not only essential, but definitely beneficial, and provided a secure environment.

Many who are not in an acute stage of illness are treated as outpatients in a hospital. Two advantages of this are that disruption to the patient's life is kept to a minimum, and the stigma attached to hospitalisation is lessened.

In some areas there are Crisis Assessment Treatment Teams (CATTs), and members of these teams will see patients in their homes. Jennifer, who has also been hospitalised, found members of these teams to be caring and emphatic individuals and said the visits were 'usually a very positive and happy experience, although at times it makes you feel so bad that you need this intensive surveillance'.

For some, however, delusional thinking during an acute manic episode has made them very aggressive and they are faced with desperate family members calling the police. Perhaps the ill person will resist the idea of a necessary stay in hospital, and may need to be certified and admitted as an involuntary patient. Being brought out of a manic episode with major tranquillisers can be an unpleasant experience not only for the patient, but also for the family members who are distressed to see a relative suffer from both the illness and from the side effects of medication.

A patient may have to face being accommodated in a closed environment, a highly stressful experience. Professor Patrick D. McGorry in *The Concept of Recovery and Secondary Prevention In Psychotic Disorders* says that in these so-called 'intensive care' units patients are accommodated in highly stimulating, frightening and intermittently dangerous environments, and cared for by staff who suffer similar stresses and risks.

Having an ill relative committed will usually be the last resort of the family because of its potential to cause fear, resentment and hostility, but family members will have to find the courage to stand firm, knowing that hospitalisation is the only way to protect a relative who has lost control and whose judgment is not sound enough to know what is needed in such a situation.

All too often, adolescents in the early stages of a psychosis are also admitted to 'intensive care' units where the most highly disturbed patients are concentrated, and this is a frightening experience for the young person suffering a first episode. Even Megan, in her thirties, whilst finding hospitalisation helpful in bringing her 'down' from a manic phase, said that her first brief stay was '... unhelpful in a lack of information and *exposure to other disturbed patients...*'

In the Western Region of Melbourne there is now an alternative for older adolescents and young adults with emerging or manifest psychotic illness. It is the Early Psychosis Prevention and Intervention Centre (EPPIC), a mental health service which aims to provide a comprehensive program of care for young people in this area and for their families. By providing effective treatment at the earliest possible stage, the program aims to minimise disruption caused, thus ensuring the best outcome for the illness itself while at the same time sustaining the young person's social, developmental and vocational interests. It has been developed in response to serious flaws in the way young people with psychotic disorders have been treated by traditional adult psychiatry services, which have been highlighted by a series of reviews, including the recent inquiry of the Human Rights Commission into the rights of the mentally ill.

A team of doctors, psychiatrists, social workers, nursing staff, psychologists, family worker and occupational therapists offer varying forms of treatment and support to patients and their families, with great emphasis on reduced disruption in social and vocational functioning, and reducing the burden and promoting the well-being of carers.

A mobile team, the Early Psychosis Assessment Team (EPAT), will provide immediate assessment and continuing information and support through each stage of assessment, in either the person's home or the local doctor's surgery or school, and respond flexibly to each situation as it presents. The Outpatient Case Management Program (OCM) then co-ordinates the patient's care to the extent of providing home-based treatment, when necessary using the 24-hour community assessment and treatment teams, while the In-Patient Unit provides care for those in need of extra support.

Families and friends are more than adequately catered for with information and personal support, and a Day Program assists individuals to maintain or re-establish a more positive personal and social role following illness.

A collaborative project with the Schizophrenia Fellowship has been established which will provide housing and support for a small group of young people in the recovery phase who have experienced homelessness or who are at significant risk.

The program began in June 1992, and indications are that delays in treatment have been reduced as young people are reached at an early stage of illness, and treatment can be commenced and managed in a more flexible and less coercive manner without having to wait for a major crisis or tragedy.

For those young people in the Western Metropolitan Region of Melbourne who are affected by psychotic illness, this discreet service, distanced from the mainstream psychiatric services, offers a sensitive and comprehensive management of their illness without the disadvantage of their being treated alongside older, more chronically disabled and disturbed patients.

The most important imminent development for EPPIC is its assistance in the establishment of a formal statewide role, which has been requested by numerous services in Victoria and interstate. EPPIC sees its role as encompassing policy input, professional education and training, development of resource materials, and other services, which would eventually result in similar services not only in Victoria, but interstate – services that would be welcomed by many needy young people and their families.

The Lord is gracious,
and full of compassion;
Slow to anger,
and of great mercy.

Psalm 145:8

11 Suicide

Suicide is frequently contemplated and sometimes carried out by depressed persons, and the issue cannot be ignored. In Australia each year, some 2500 people commit suicide, choosing death over life, and 60 000 attempt it. Of these, around seventy per cent have a depressive illness. The real figures may be actually higher than this, because many single-car accidents are considered attempted or actual suicides. Twice as many women as men attempt suicide, but men succeed more often.

The reasons for suicide are generally not well understood within the community, or even by the individual's family and friends. Those left behind will go through a period of deep and painful soul-searching, trying to find the answers. 'Could I have done something to prevent it?' 'Did I ignore the warning signs?' 'Did I fail to listen?' 'Why didn't I realise he was so depressed?'

Those further removed from a suicide will often have a different set of statements. 'Why did he do it?' 'How could she leave the little ones like that — it's so selfish.' 'She had everything to live for.' 'I just don't understand!' I've even heard it said, with a tinge of horror, 'If she was *that* depressed surely she could have had a good cry ... talked with someone!' The crux of the matter is that people do not understand, because as a whole we are not educated in this area. The popular reaction to suicide is always disbelief, and often the judgment of selfishness and weakness of character. It must surely be the most misunderstood act, and such judgment is pronounced by people who have never been touched by the preceding anguish and pain. Stigma should not be attached to suicide victims who are, after all, victims of a crippling illness, especially when euthanasia is supported by so many for victims of other illnesses.

Many believe the myth: 'If he talks about it, he won't do it. He's just seeking attention.' This is a most dangerous myth. Many depressed people *don't* want help, because they firmly believe their situation is beyond help. They actually believe death is their only solution. All suicidal thoughts and actions should be taken very seriously, particularly if they have occurred previously.

People who talk about the hopelessness of their situation, and warn that they can see no solution other than suicide, may toy with the idea for some time, perhaps attempting and failing with different methods until they find the method that suits them.

Suicide is usually the act of a person who is confused and despairing, and who sees no hope at all for the future. To distorted thinking, suicide is a rational solution. If you suspect someone near you is contemplating 'putting an end to it all', try to get him or her to professional help immediately. In the meantime, just talking can bring relief. The idea that his or her life is too precious to throw away may not persuade sufficiently, because of distorted thinking. This person already believes his or her life is not worth saving. Emphasise the effect the death will have on loved ones. Say how you will feel when he or she is no longer there. Many people talking of suicide don't really want to die, when it's all said and done. They just want an end to their pain, and may appreciate the opportunity to reconsider.

By the same token, many others act on their impulse quickly and unexpectedly, so if the suicidal person is a relative or friend being treated for depression, call the treating psychiatrist immediately, as hospitalisation may be necessary.

Most people who commit suicide are depressed. Aaron T. Beck in his book *Depression: Causes and Treatment* says that, in one study, suicidal wishes were present in approximately one-third of individuals with a mild case of depression, and in nearly three-quarters of people who were severely depressed. He also said that, in the USA, it had been estimated that the number of depressed people who die as a result of suicide is approximately twenty-five times the suicide rate within the general population.

Suicides, or attempted suicides, in depressed people, unlike many others, do not contain the elements of aggression, hate or revenge. Rather, death promises relief from suffering, a suffering that includes the unshakable conviction that one is not worthy of life and too great a burden for one's family to bear. Often it appears to be the only logical solution if these people sincerely believe that:

- there is no hope for the future (feelings of hopelessness have set in)
- they will never again be anything but a hindrance to those around them
- they will never again be well
- they cannot bear any more suffering
- they are so worthless or bad that death is a suitable punishment

As they sink lower into the depths of depression, it is important to remember that the mind is capable only of dwelling on the darkness of the present and all the bad things in the past. They are unable to see any happiness, past or present, and unable to imagine a future, let alone any future happiness, and suicidal thoughts become more and more pervasive as they lose all hope for an end to pain. This is a concept that most individuals are simply unable to comprehend.

Spike Milligan, recognising the difficulty that other people experience, explains it this way:

> Only when you know what it is like to feel depressed, to feel you are dying inside, can you know what it is like to be suicidal, to think that the whole dreadful, terrible, nagging, awful pain of it all might be swept away by a simple, single act of self-destruction.

At times, the extreme dullness of mind and sluggishness of body may make it difficult to actually carry out the act. It is often when the depression appears to have lifted and the person seems quite tranquil that the suicide occurs, because this is the time when he or she has the energy and initiative needed to carry out the act as planned.

At that time, having made the decision, a great peace of mind may be experienced because the burden of life has suddenly been lifted, but unfortunately, others will be so deceived by his or her demeanour that they will not be expecting the act of suicide.

There was a time when I lost all hope of my ongoing depression ever lifting, and I reached for my bottles of pills. But I knew, looking at them, that there were not enough, and I also knew that my present life, no matter how bad it seemed, was better than swallowing too few pills and ending up so physically ill that I was an even bigger burden on my family. There were a number of times when I felt so low that thoughts of death constantly flooded my mind, and I often rang the local psychiatric hospital or Lifeline, sometimes in the middle of the night, hoping that someone could snap me out of my wretchedness.

Deep down I did not want to die, but I could see no other way out, and I really believed that I might suddenly take that final step in desperation. There was always a measure of comfort in hearing the understanding professional voice, not exactly breaking through my wall of darkness but at least trying. I was always reminded that I had come through bouts like this before and I would again, and no matter what I thought, my family did need me. How would my daughters feel if I ended my life this way? Maybe I didn't agree, but I did listen, and it gave me something to cling to throughout the night.

Then came my blackest moment, when I lost all hope. I knew that I could no longer look after my daughters, knew that I could not expect them to want to live with such a poor excuse for a mother. The only sensible solution was to leave them permanently, let them get on with their lives, free of me and my illness. What use is a woman too ill to look after herself, always letting family and friends down?

As soon as my mood lifted sufficiently, I did carry out the necessary research into which pills to take and how many, and made a new will in readiness. But, following a rapid lift in mood and a visit to my doctor, I again saw some hope for the future and decided to shelve my plan at that stage. However, the predominant reason for my capitulation was that I finally had a choice. There was a sense of freedom in having a method worked out to end it all, knowing that I no longer had to be dominated by my moods.

When I was in a somewhat better frame of mind, I told my husband what I had done and where my will was. He told me that I was very selfish, and he made me realise that the girls would carry long-term emotional scars if I left them in such a gruesome manner. As he said, 'It's better to have a mentally ill mother than no mother at all'. But my irrational mind had been contemplating the act with their welfare in mind.

Still somewhat depressed, I forced myself to contemplate the question of suicide from my daughters' point of view. They would be left to deal with a huge legacy of pain and unjustified guilt, and it now caused me great anguish to think that I had almost brought this down on their young shoulders. I dwelt on the grief my daughters would bear, trying to make it a fixed part of my thinking, to help me cope with the next bout of depression. I even typed the words, with a short prayer, on a small slip of paper and kept it in my bedside drawer, looking at it from time to time.

That little slip of paper is still in my bedside drawer, to remind me of the darkness that temporarily blinded me, and the happiness I rediscovered when I was again able to accept life over death. I learned from that episode that no matter how deep our despair, it can be eased if we seek and accept help, or if help is offered. We all need help in weathering these storms, and we must always remember that they *do* pass.

There is another aspect to suicide we never see, never talk about. Suicide is often portrayed in movies as a fairly quick, clean and painless act. In fact it isn't. It is usually very messy and is never the painless release that is expected. Many, in their clumsy attempts, end up alive but brain-damaged, or they die much later on, suffering an agonising death from internal injuries or infection. The very real picture of suicide is often a body disfigured by pain, perhaps drowning in its own vomit, or choking on its tongue, and it is a tragedy that a person's suffering can lead to such an end. Suicide is never pretty, and many people must surely have second thoughts when it is too late. Life, no matter how bleak, no matter how painful the future looks, must surely be difficult to relinquish as a person crosses the boundary into the unknown.

I once talked with a man who refused to go to his friend's funeral because that friend had committed suicide. He thought it a 'stupid thing to do'. He could not reach out to try to learn something of his friend's circumstances, to better understand why he had taken that drastic step. Had he been able to, it might have eased his own grief and bitterness.

Compassion is the appropriate response for those who attempt or commit suicide.

The community in general needs to be better educated about suicide and needs to try to gain an understanding of why people choose death over life.

Many funeral companies now offer community education programs for pastoral and community care workers. Tobin Brothers of Melbourne, because they believe that suicide is possibly the most confronting of all deaths, provides a seminar titled 'Responding to the Survivors of Suicide' which covers the myths, facts and impact of suicide, the messages given to the survivors by society, and the care of the survivors. In so doing, they are helping to ensure not only that the survivors receive necessary counselling, but that ultimately the community in general is being better informed.

Their representatives also work with teachers and counsellors about death and grieving, with aspects of suicide also being incorporated if requested. This must surely be beneficial to upper secondary school children, in light of the drug problems and turmoil so prevalent in this age group, and the fact that many of them will already have encountered at least one person who has had to grapple with the pain of a friend's suicide, attempted suicide, or serious thoughts about suicide.

The Directorate of School Education, Melbourne, has a school support service responsible for the counselling of children in crisis, including those who have encountered, contemplated or attempted suicide. Where depression or other worrying signs are noticed in a student, school welfare co-ordinators can provide initial support and, if further assistance is deemed necessary, the student will be seen by either a directorate-employed social worker, or a guidance officer who is teacher-trained with experience in schools and qualified as a psychologist. If that person encounters suicidal tendencies or manic-depressive illness in a student, the student can be referred, in discussion with the parents, to Community Services or a doctor or psychiatrist, either through the public or private system.

Ms Glenda Johnston of the Directorate of School Education in Melbourne chaired a Youth Suicide Reference Group comprising social workers and guidance officers throughout the state, and their aims were, and remain, to discuss all issues that need attention, and the resources available, and to draw the threads of both areas together so that the system provides the best possible care for youth in need of special assistance. A Youth Suicide Working Party containing representatives from the Catholic, independent and State education systems as well as leading psychiatrists, Health and Community Services representatives, the Coroner and other interest groups, recognises that depression is an area of very real concern and has been looking at ways of bettering the methods of dealing with the problem. Special note has been taken of the results of a survey of the health of all secondary school students by the Centre for Adolescent Health, which confirmed a very high level of depression amongst adolescents.

The Austin Hospital in Melbourne conducts a program called Homelessness Agency Resource Program (HARP), the aim of which is suicide prevention in youth. Under this program, which has now been running successfully for several years, housing workers who work with homeless youth are trained by professional staff in the area of suicide prevention.

There have also been various other studies that look into the causes of suicide, and preventative measures to be taken, particularly in relation to youth, one such study being that undertaken by the Victorian State Coroner.

The television campaign recently run by the Federal Government to promote understanding of mental illness will, by its very nature, also save lives because people will, hopefully, adopt a more understanding, compassionate and caring attitude, which can only be of benefit to sufferers of mental illness.

Clearly, there is a move towards gaining an insight into why people, particularly the young, attempt suicide, and ultimately this will lead to a lessening of the incidence. But families of severely depressed people need to be better educated, and people who are suicidally depressed should be asked by their doctor or therapist to confront their suicidal ideas, to face the practicalities of the act and look at the alternatives. Suicidal thoughts should be brought out into the open, not treated lightly or ignored. It must be recognised that the depressed person has a great need to talk about these thoughts.

Suicide is forever, not just for the victim, but for those left behind. The better alternative is to accept help and choose life.

There are many myths that the families of depressed persons should be aware of, among them being:

Myth: People who talk about suicide do not commit suicide.

Fact: Talkers are often doers and threats should be taken seriously.

Myth: Suicide happens without warning.

Fact: Potential suicides often make threats. Often the more specific the threat, the greater the probability of a serious attempt.

Myth: Suicidal people are fully intent on dying.

Fact: Many appreciate the opportunity to reconsider. They are only looking for an end to their pain.

Myth: Once a person is suicidal, he or she is suicidal forever.

Fact: They often find ways to strengthen their resolve to live and go on to lead happy and productive lives.

Myth: Improvement following a suicidal crisis means the risk is over.

Fact: The mood change from suicidal depression to apparent tranquillity may in fact reflect that a person has made the decision to commit suicide, and the tranquillity is merely the result of feeling the burden lifted.

Myth: Suicide strikes more often amongst the rich, or almost exclusively among the poor.

Fact: It is not confined to any one group within the community.

God, teach me to be patient –
Teach me to go slow –
Teach me how to 'wait on You'
When my way I do not know …

Helen Steiner Rice

12 Family and friends

Family

Manic-depressive illness has a particularly disruptive effect on the sufferer's family. Not only will they have to maintain their responsibilities at work and school, and other commitments outside the home, but they will now have to share an additional workload in the home and help in the care and management of the ill relative. At the same time they have to contend with their feelings of embarrassment, frustration, fear, anger or guilt.

If the ill person happens to be young, parents have to endure the additional distress of watching their child suffer, often wishing they could change places. Suddenly, the child's school or job prospects must be put on hold, and the future is unknown and uncertain. The family's own future hopes and plans will also have to be held in abeyance; this often causes anger and guilt.

Siblings face their own particular problems too. No longer is there any fun in the household. All the parents' time and attention is going towards the sick child, and money could be more scarce because of medical and pharmaceutical bills. Siblings may have feelings of guilt because, deep down, they're relieved they did not develop the illness, but they may fear for their own future offspring.

Marriages are under enormous strain. If one partner is ill, then the other loses that person for the time being. If it is a child, the parents expend so much time and energy on caring for the child that they have little left for each other. It is most important for family members to look after their own physical and mental well-being. A bit of 'time out' on a regular basis does wonders, as does joining a support group or other organisation for carers or relatives and friends, where they can meet people in the same situation. These groups offer education, assistance in many areas including accommodation, crisis services and counselling, information on a wide range of issues, friendship, emotional support, counselling and support by way of telephone services, newsletters, professional guest speakers at meetings, library and video services. Then, when the lives of the family members have settled down in the future, they in turn may well be able to help others.

Children of an ill parent can also find themselves in embarrassing situations, particularly if the parent is manic. My daughter suffered great personal humiliation during one episode, listening to me chat with her friends about the prospect of my heading off to a disco.

Unfortunately, the warning signs of a high are often so intangible that the person is caught up in it without being aware, and once in that state is often so headstrong that others don't quite know how to handle it. With mild swings in particular it can be very difficult to know at just what point normal mood is left behind and disordered mood begins. With a first episode, family members do not understand what is happening, nor how to deal with it, so confusion is rife. It is then imperative to seek professional help as quickly as possible.

The next step is for the family members to become well informed about the illness, its course and treatment, side effects of the medication, and how they can each participate in the treatment program. They should also be aware of the signs that warn of an impending episode so that treatment can be modified if necessary to prevent or lessen its effects.

Relatives should be aware, however, that with a first episode the psychiatrist may not immediately be able to give a precise diagnosis and prognosis. In certain cases it may take time to determine whether the person is suffering from manic-depressive illness or schizophrenia because of certain similarities and, even when a diagnosis of manic-depressive illness can be confirmed, it is not possible to say at the outset what the course of the illness will be. As we know, many people recover quickly and do not have a further relapse, whilst others may have fluctuations over a long period of time. Psychiatrists and medical staff often fear presenting too optimistic or pessimistic an outlook, as either way both patient and relatives stand to suffer. But many families, in the midst of a crisis and not understanding what is happening, expect immediate answers and hope for an instant cure.

Unfortunately, the world of psychiatry is not as clearly defined as that of general medicine where a broken leg can be set in plaster and an infection treated with antibiotics. Many of the respondents to my questionnaire were not correctly diagnosed for months and, in some cases years (in the latter cases, most of the initial diagnoses were made some twenty years ago before the more recent development of reliable diagnostic systems).

These illnesses are very intrusive, and as symptoms are manifested, particularly with hypomania and mania, the relatives will often feel enormous shame, not wanting neighbours and friends to know there is mental illness in the family. Each family member will learn to deal with the necessary adjustments in his or her own way. At times, particularly in the initial stages or when the symptoms are not too severe, some will deny the fact of mental illness, attributing the swings in mood to external causes or personality traits. But if the illness persists and the symptoms become severe, they will have to give it due recognition and attention. The more quickly the family are able to pull together in an atmosphere of knowledge and unanimity, the easier it will be for everyone.

This is where family counselling can be invaluable. Among other things, families need to learn that the depressed person feels very fatigued, becomes quite emotionless, and will usually respond negatively to their well-intentioned approaches; that in mania the reckless and energetic behaviour can be tiring, embarrassing, even frightening. In family counselling, family members all come together with a counsellor or therapist and are able to air their problems and concerns so that coping strategies can be worked out, both to help the family understand and deal with the effects of the illness, and to deal with their own fluctuating emotions. This can be particularly helpful if the sufferer is an adolescent struggling for independence, perhaps rejecting the need for medication and resenting what he or she sees as parental interference.

Liz, mother of 22-year-old Emma who suffers from manic-depression, finds the day-to-day management of her daughter's illness very difficult, wishing she could truly understand her daughter's awful, mysterious world. Liz says:

> As a family we have moved from feeling sorry for ourselves about living with this totally different family member who disrupts and confuses everyone's lives – to one of such great love and relief that we aren't going through *her* experience. But even so, it's 'tuff' being so understanding.

The grief and loss of our 'real Emma' is hard too, but ... I put those thoughts behind me and deal with the Emma I live with *now* (not yesterday).

Depressed people find it very difficult to communicate to their family how they feel, not wanting to be any more of a burden than they already are. They withdraw, filled with guilt and self-loathing because they feel they are failing their family. And the family members, not fully understanding what is happening to their loved one, and often feeling tired and depressed themselves, might try to cajole him or her out of the mood, or become insistent that life cannot possibly be *that* bad, thus adding to the load of guilt.

It is very distressing to watch the family unit being torn apart by this illness, but it is very important that there be someone within the family circle who is prepared to offer quiet and positive encouragement and to just listen at times. The value of the art of listening cannot be underestimated for a depressed person. Many family members become so bogged down in their pain that, for their self-preservation, they either try to switch off emotionally, or become too forceful in trying to bring about a change of mood in their loved one.

Being able to act calmly is enormously valuable, particularly if the ill person becomes aggressive, which is usually due to fear or uncontrollable emotions. It may help to remember that he or she was not always that way and certainly does not enjoy being that way.

The other side of the coin is that, at times, the person should be helped to become aware of what the family has endured, particularly through manic episodes, and should be asked to consider ways in which the family's difficulties can be minimised. An example would be my own case, where I had overloaded all my credit cards whilst high, and I was asked to either hand them over to my husband or cut them up.

If it is the wife and mother who is ill, the time may come when the husband has to take over the management of the household. Unfortunately, this may initially cause the woman a lot of extra guilt, but if the husband remains calm and reassures her that it is only a temporary situation, her anxiety will soon pass and she will benefit enormously by being relieved of the burden of impossible decision-making and having to perform beyond her capability.

Even when the person is experiencing normal mood, there can be problems. When there has been a number of hypomanic or manic episodes, the family can become very eagle-eyed, suspicious of every comment or action that rings a warning bell. This can put a strain on the natural ebb and flow of the ill person's actions and emotions. If the person wants to go shopping, her or his mood is instantly called into question. If he or she wants to go out with friends one evening, not having done so for a long time, again motives are questioned. The family is naturally anxious, often causing the person to feel stifled and resentful if constantly made to answer for every move while mood is normal. It is difficult for everyone, but again family counselling will help to work out strategies best suited to the particular needs of the family.

Family members should know the doctor's telephone number should an emergency arise, and the medications the person is taking, the dosages, and where the medications are kept. It can also be helpful, in case of an accident outside the home, if the ill person wears a *medical alert bracelet* which contains all personal details together with details of medications, allergies to particular medications, blood type, and so on. This is important when medication should not be brought to an abrupt halt, or where an allergy has developed to a particular medication, such as penicillin.

Under no circumstances should family or friends advise the ill person to discontinue medication. Watching a person swallowing pills morning and night, particularly when side effects are visible, is a constant and irritating reminder that life is not as we would like, and it can be tempting to suggest that medication be stopped. But severe depression can quickly lead to a suicide attempt, and mania or hypomania also have the potential for great disaster such as reckless, uninhibited, even dangerous behaviour, or the spending of huge sums of money.

Friends

Friends also have a difficult and important role to play. In the initial stages, they flounder for answers along with everyone else, and they too may take the road of denial until symptoms become so prolonged and severe that the illness can no longer be denied.

In the case of a middle-aged person, friends might conclude that it is a 'mid-life crisis' or menopause, and in the case of a young person it might be put down to the usual teenage turmoil. As the months roll by, friends will accept the situation but find it very disconcerting. They may not know how to handle their friend, or what to say, and their efforts to help may seem to be falling on deaf ears.

Those who have never encountered mental illness (and this is the majority) are afraid of what they don't understand, afraid too because they recognise the complexities and frailties of their own minds, and it is difficult to be brought face to face with those frailties.

The manic-depressive sufferer can cause personal embarrassment by outrageous behaviour during a hypomanic or manic episode, particularly when out in company. I have seen the looks of discomfort, and later have felt my own brand of humiliation following an episode when I've unwittingly embarrassed a friend. A long-standing friend may tolerate this sort of behaviour, may even deal with it calmly, but not everyone has that capacity.

During depression, of course, the ill person will withdraw from friends, discontinuing all associations, and the situation is often exacerbated when panic attacks occur and social engagements are broken.

Friends become confused by the erratic behaviour that mood swings bring, and many will drift away, feeling rejected, betrayed or hurt. Some do not have the necessary strength or commitment to take on the additional burden of such a friendship.

Norma Farnes, a friend of Spike Milligan, found that many of his friends stayed away – a few stayed in touch, but some, she said, were just too embarrassed. In *Depression and How to Survive It* Norma summed it up this way:

> You say 'Spike is not well' and they say 'Oh Dear!' What the fuck does that mean, 'Oh Dear'? You know I never hear people saying 'Is there anything we can do?'

Spike himself described it this way:

> When I was first ill no-one seemed to notice. I was screaming inside, hurting and hoping someone would do something. Maybe I would have told them to mind their own business but I don't think so. I think I would have said 'Thank God'.

Norma Farnes pointed out:

> Well they might ring him up and just listen to him. He needs people. All you have to do is go upstairs and sit with him, hold his hand. He needs people. He needs to know that there is someone there. Because he feels so alone. He feels, or at least I think he feels that he is not well and that only he can cope with it. The truth is, however, that he actually cannot cope with it and in the early stages he only copes by screaming and shouting.

When asked how an understanding person might cope with a depressed friend, Spike responded, 'Immediately he'll reach out emotionally and say "What can I do to help? Let me sit and talk to you a while".'

From the sufferer's point of view, when mood returns to normal, it can be soul-destroying to step back into reality only to discover that one's friendships have suffered what appears at the time to be irreparable damage.

Megan says that the effects on her social life were devastating.

Friends found my extreme depression hard to be around. I was asked to leave a house I was sharing with one friend and that led to virtually leaving one group of friends entirely. I had been very gregarious, and my depression seemed to raise an acute sense of loneliness and insecurity. I was afraid of being alone, and the sense of being abandoned by my friends made my life a torment. Several friends seemed to believe that 'I could pull myself out of it if I wanted to'; that I could control my mood. Various ones became impatient, angry and, I felt, disdainful of me. One friend said simply 'Depressed people aren't fun to be with'. I guess they aren't.

It left me trying to find new accommodation and companions at a time when I felt least able to do it. It was easier for friends who did not see me so frequently; they remained supportive.

It was at that time I was referred to ARAFEMI (Association of Relatives and Friends of the Emotionally and Mentally Ill) and found a group of people who understood what I was going through and accepted me as I was.

Not surprisingly, people emerging from depression can experience extreme loneliness. They feel the need to be involved in something meaningful and productive, to be appreciated, but when the friends are gone and perhaps the job too, or even family members, it is easy to become discouraged and bewildered and lapse into depression and anxiety again. As Angela Rossmanith says in *The Self Alone*:

... When there is little or no emotional support available, the ability to cope with setbacks or personal difficulties is limited; accordingly, resistance to feelings of despair is weakened, and suicide may seem the only option, ...

... It is up to all of us to try to read the signs: when we work on deeper levels of contact and understanding we have a better chance of recognising someone who is in need of help.

The sense of loneliness that emerges when relative stability is regained can be considered a sign of better health, vastly different from the feeling of isolation experienced during depression. It can be a sign of renewed life, and should be accepted as such. It is the time to experience normal emotions, work through them with help and support, and rebuild on the foundations of old friendships or, if necessary, to make a fresh start with new friends.

I have often thought that a true friendship is like a solid house. We lay a strong foundation on which we build, brick by brick, until it provides shelter, warmth, and protection from life's storms. Over the years a few cracks will appear and be patched up. If the cracks are left to widen, eventually the walls may crumble, but still the foundation will remain, and if it was strong enough, can be rebuilt upon.

Many friendships can be renewed, and the new bond is often stronger than ever. Often the old friends were merely waiting in the wings for the performer to finish the act.

How family and friends can help

People living with a depressed person for any length of time often end up feeling depressed themselves, because nothing they do or say seems to make any difference. There's no magic answer to depression, but the following very helpful suggestions have been adapted from the MD Papers of the Depressive and Manic Depressive Association of NSW:

- **Reassure** that the depression will end – over and over. Depressed people cannot see the light at the end of the tunnel, and need this reassurance. Although they might say that they don't believe it, it does help to hear that things will improve.

- **Work out a program** to combat the depression. One of the horrible aspects of depression is a sense of powerlessness. Working out a program can help restore a feeling of slowly getting control again. Things to combat depression might be as varied as planning not to be alone, exercise, extra vitamins, medication, doing pleasant things as often as possible. Just getting out of bed in the morning could be a good start.

- **Remove guilt**. Depressed people feel guilty about everything from being born to being depressed right now. Guilt is a symptom of depression just as much as the slowness and crying are symptoms. Tell the person that you understand: 'It's a treatable illness.' 'It's not your fault.' 'There is no need for you to feel bad about your performance as partner/parent/friend.' Don't make the person feel guilty about taking drugs – depression is a biochemical condition and often needs medication; it's not a sign of moral failure.

- **Encourage but don't push.** Ever tried climbing a mountain with every step a moment of agony, anguish, pain? Even the simplest task can seem insurmountable to someone who's depressed. Encourage and reassure: 'You *can* do it.' 'It doesn't matter if it is not perfect.' Help to break the task up into manageable bits, rewarding any small attempts: 'You and I both know what you can do when you are well; it's great that you have managed to do this when you are depressed.'

- **Treat any threat of suicide seriously.** Many people might not want to die; they just want to stop existing in this horrible state of mind, or kill off just that depressed worthless part of themselves. Seek help promptly if you suspect someone is planning to give it all up. Talks about suicide with another person do help. When the suicidal thoughts come up they can be stopped by thinking of positive thoughts put forward by another person. Talking of suicide can be a 'nothing is working, what's the point' cry for help. Talking it through should include practical ways of coping with the thoughts, such as not being on one's own, keeping drugs out of the way to avoid any temptation to blot it all out, and reassessing appropriate medication. Thinking positive thoughts about living, such as 'just waiting for my daughter's birthday next month' or 'seeing the moon rise just one more time' might be enough to avert this crisis.

- **Care for your own life.** Depression is contagious, so ensure that your life is pleasant, fulfilling and not being badly affected by someone close not wanting to go out or have people visit. It will only generate guilt if you restrict your life too. Would your partner/friend be happier sleeping than painfully trying to cope with a party? Decide how much help you are prepared and able to give, and try not to be resentful if your help seems unappreciated; enjoy your own life.

The treating psychiatrist should always be contacted when a manic or hypomanic episode manifests itself, as medication may need to be reassessed and altered, and hospitalisation may be necessary. Symptoms to watch for include the following:

- sleeplessness for several nights
- irritable, aggressive, or threatening mood
- increased socialisation
- reckless spending or impulsive decisions
- pressured speech

Because the mood can shift quickly from euphoria to irritability, even aggression, and because there is a great potential for sexual indiscretions and overspending, the family should act quickly. Again, it is helpful if there is one member of the family who accepts responsibility for recognising the symptoms and alerting the ill relative to the fact that help must be sought, because he or she often does not recognise that anything is wrong, insisting that the situation is quite normal. Usually, who takes on this role will have been discussed in consultation with the treating psychiatrist, and agreed to by the ill person as part of a formulated plan to (a) reduce the need for hospitalisation, (b) reduce the risk of unacceptable behaviour, and (c) place a limit on the strain endured by the family.

Obviously it becomes somewhat easier for the family to cope once they have learned to recognise the signs of an impending swing, and once they are aware of the situations and topics of conversation that tend to trigger aggression and unacceptable behaviour, which can then often be avoided, using the strategies already worked out with the psychiatrist or health care worker, or in family counselling.

Becoming angry in such circumstances is unhelpful. It is always preferable to remain calm and, if your pleas to your relative to seek help are being ignored, you can yourself make contact with the treating psychiatrist or hospital.

Help for the family

There are many organisations available to families these days which provide counselling, support, friendship, referral to appropriate services and, above all, a sympathetic ear for those really bad times. Some of these organisations are listed in the resource section at the back of this book.

The importance of the roles played by support groups, both in the areas of emotional and educational support, and in consumerism and advocacy, has been stressed extensively throughout the book *Families of the Mentally Ill*, in which Agnes P. Hatfield and Harriet P. Lefley have brought together a professionally diverse group of people from the areas of psychology, education, nursing, psychiatry and rehabilitation, who write with the aim of focusing on the family and how it experiences the tragedy of mental illness in a loved one. Hatfield and Lefley hope to provide mental health professionals with a better understanding of mental illness from a family perspective.

The book is directed at mental health professionals and contains comprehensive information based on extensive research in many areas including culture, behavioural manifestations of mental illness, the meaning of mental illness to the family (including the extended family), the evolution of family responses to mental illness through time, social support and family coping, coping strategies of family caregivers, and much more.

Despite the fact that it is written for professionals, it provides such an in-depth look into areas such as behavioural problems and helpful strategies that readers will readily identify with the situations illustrated and should gain a deeper insight into their own situation and be able to benefit from the suggested methods of dealing with common problems. One chapter is devoted to the pattern of family responses, or the manner in which families work their way through ten suggested stages, starting with ignorance and shock, later searching for causes and treatment, then collapse of optimism, mourning the loss of the idealised internal images of the ill person, and ultimately picking up the pieces and restoring balance in the lives of the family members.

The book is well worth reading, even though it may prove more demanding than other books that have been less extensively researched.

Of the many thousands of carers in Australia, large numbers have had to put their own hopes, dreams and careers on hold. The important role played by these people has finally been given due recognition during the past four to five years, with large studies and research projects being conducted in an effort to ascertain firstly, the experiences and needs of carers, and secondly, the best ways of reducing the burden and poor health experienced by carers.

One such comprehensive research project, undertaken by the University of Melbourne and funded by the Health Promotion Foundation, began in 1989. One anticipated recommendation is for a specific person in a hospital to be designated as the 'family worker'. This person's role would be to approach the family or caregivers of each person admitted to the hospital with a view to providing any necessary assistance.

The Carers Program, with the help of the Australian Institute of Family Studies, has conducted a state-wide random telephone survey of over 1000 carers across Victoria, the aim of the research team being to build a true picture of informal caregiving in a variety of situations and geographic locations, survey findings being used to develop strategies for assisting carers and to provide the basis for recommendations to changes in social policy according to carers' needs. It was revealed in the pilot study that serious health problems exist among family carers, and that there is a very low usage of community services.

Children who have a parent suffering from major mental illness have also been targeted in another research study by the Early Psychosis Research Centre. Information gathered included numbers of such children, the supports families are able to use, and whether or not those supports are being accessed. The aim is for the information to be used to acquaint family and psychiatric services with any gaps that exist, and to suggest programs that will effectively support children and give workers in a wide range of settings additional information to support the families with whom they work.

In an age when the responsibility of care and management of the ill person rests with the family more than ever before, it is most heartening to know that the dedication of carers and the hardships they endure are being recognised, and that associated problems and needs are being addressed.

The Federal Government has also recognised the important role that a carer plays and the necessity of having a working partnership between carers and health professionals. To assist carers to tap into avenues of support, it has produced a kit called 'Carer Support: Practical Information on Caring at Home', which contains fact sheets covering areas such as Carer Emergency Plan, How to Care Safely at Home, Audio Tape featuring Carers Talk, and Carer's Relaxation. Copies of the kit can be obtained from the Carers Association in each state by using the telephone numbers and addresses provided at the back of this book.

Many of the organisations listed in this book are also able to provide accommodation for the ill, and this service can prove to be a necessary and invaluable aid for many people.

Knowing that the plight of carers is being investigated should comfort some families, who would find it in their best interests to join one of the available organisations where their voices can be heard. Above all, family members should never lose heart. Manic-depressive illness is episodic and, although at times it may seem unyielding to all attempts to control it, there will be an end to each episode, and the ill person will revert to normal mood.

After the clouds, the sunshine,
After the winter, the spring,
After the shower, the rainbow –
For life is a changeable thing.

Helen Steiner Rice

13 Coming full circle

Eventually we come full circle. Having weathered the storms, most of us will eventually be stabilised on maintenance medication and can start, little by little, to take our lives into our own hands again, leaving behind the burden of guilt and despair we have carried around for so long. For some, there will have been one or two episodes, for others many ups and downs.

We do not suddenly become well again and stay well forever more. Even when stabilised, there are often fluctuations that call for adjustments in medication, and for many this process lasts for some time. The important things to remember are that you should know your own illness and take responsibility for the management of it, and you should respect any pain and fatigue and learn how to live and deal with it. Listen to your body. If it tells you to rest a while, then take some time out. Additional rest one day can mean greater achievement and satisfaction the next.

As periods of normal mood become more frequent, you may be uncertain of which thoughts, feelings and behaviour are normal and which stem from any mild fluctuations you may be experiencing. This can be a very frustrating period, and you may withdraw periodically because you lack confidence. Observe and try to identify your feelings and reactions. I can highly recommend keeping a journal as a tool to deal with emotional upheaval, regaining self-esteem and confidence, and setting future goals. You need only the ability to conduct a dialogue with yourself and write it down. It has enormous therapeutic value. By writing down your thoughts, you are becoming more aware of how your thought processes work and how they govern your emotional and behavioural responses. If you have started a journal during the period of your illness, you are also providing a means of measuring your progress.

Once you are stabilised, it is important to set goals for yourself: small goals at first, ones you know you can achieve. It may be just a short walk each day to improve your level of fitness, or to catch up with friends you have neglected due to illness. Later on it may be taking up a hobby or a short course of study. Some days when you're feeling really down, it may be just getting out of bed, taking a shower and making a cup of tea. It doesn't matter what the goal, as long as you make a conscious decision and act on it. And when you have successes, be sure to record them in the journal. Without the sense of purpose that accompanies goal-setting, your new-found life of stability may seem empty at first, and you may feel unfulfilled, which could very quickly lead to anxiety and depression.

Do not let well-meaning relatives and friends set unrealistic goals for you. Because you appear to be so much better now, they tend to forget that there may be constant fluctuations for some time to come. Listen to their suggestions, but accept only what you know you are capable of achieving.

For many there will still be wearying battles along the way. Relationships may have been shattered, family life disrupted, careers and jobs lost, and on top of all that, self-esteem and confidence will have been severely eroded.

Even after years of suffering, many try to keep the knowledge of their illness from friends, because they fear the stigma attached to it. We have all felt this at one time or another, heard the sniggers or whispers, been refused employment or been dismissed from a job. But we should concentrate on patient and family education in managing the illness, and public education in understanding, so that discrimination is lessened; we should keep our heads high, draw comfort from those who love us, and accept judgment only from God.

Often when we have come through a shattering ordeal, our faith in our deity, in life itself, has been crushed. We may have reached the point of believing that we will never have any peace of mind, any happiness. We still feel quite desperate, not knowing which way to turn, but any residual feelings of pain or fear will soon be tempered by new feelings of lightness and peace, because we have been relieved of our great burden. Even in the midst of pain and confusion, happiness exists within us, if only as a seed waiting for nourishment. We must find and nurture the seed and it will flourish and grow, even alongside any unpleasantness that may come our way.

On a more practical note, at this time you might still have physical, mental, emotional and spiritual readjustments to make, so it would be wise to seek counselling from your psychiatrist, therapist, and/or religious minister with whom you can discuss any of these residual problems. Support groups can also be very helpful.

It is possible that some of us will slip back a few paces from time to time, again making us wonder if the end is really in sight. We may feel overwhelmed by a sense of failure if we do not handle this well, but remember that it will pass, as all other bad spells have passed, and we will again move forward with renewed strength.

With this illness I discovered a fortitude that I would never have believed possible, and I gained the confidence and courage to be true to myself. I no longer rely so heavily on the approval of others for my self-esteem, and I now make choices that are right for my needs. I have learned not to be such a perfectionist, and not to impose unrealistic expectations on myself. Peace of mind and self-worth are now valued more highly.

I am learning to give of myself again as I rediscover love and understanding, compassion and tolerance, and there is a new pleasure in rediscovering simple things such as participating in family life, coffee with a friend, or going for a walk. Above all, every moment of good health, composure and sanity is treasured.

While I have learned to accept my illness, I will always treat it with respect, aware that I may falter along the way from time to time, that it is controlled, not cured. I also recognise the fact that each year has continued to show a steady improvement in my general health.

Those whom I have not told will not know of my illness unless they hear it from my lips or read my book, because my behaviour is usually no different from that of any person working in the same position as I do, and I rarely suffer such diminished capacity in my ability to perform what is expected of me that I have to take time away from work. Although I consider myself to be quite stable, my mood can still fluctuate up to twenty per cent above or below normal, which means that I have to try just a little harder than the average person to present a normal face to the world, but I do not consider this challenge too difficult.

Some people are not in such a fortunate position. They may have lost their jobs in the early stages of illness, lost their skills and confidence, ended up joining the lengthy dole queue, unemployable, and have lost all self-esteem. This is not a good menu for them to try to begin a new life, because the new day will hold no light, no hope. However, as long as the illness has improved, even marginally, support and counselling can restore some degree of motivation and hope. Improvement can be achieved, just one step at a time. Goals must start off being simple. It is useless to jump in at the deep end and expect miracles to happen. Re-training in something less stressful for the unemployed can be of great value, but again this is where counselling is necessary.

There are also the people whose illness has other complications, and they spend more time in hospital that out in the world. They may live in community housing, without family, or have families who do not want to know them, who cannot cope with the illness. Such circumstances make it even more difficult, almost impossible, for them to progress from total dependence on their psychiatrist or health worker to living any sort of life in the normal sense.

I would like to end on a more positive note. For those with spiritual beliefs there is always the knowledge when emerging from illness that we are no longer alone. We are no longer chained in the dark abyss, alone, in pain and desperation. We can rely on One stronger than ourselves who watches over us in all our misery and in our recovery.

> One night I dreamed a dream.
> I was walking along the beach
> with my Lord.
> Across the dark sky flashed scenes
> from my life.
> For each scene, I noticed two sets
> of footprints in the sand,
> one belonging to me
> and one to my Lord.
> When the last scene of my life
> shot before me
> I looked back at the footprints in the
> sand.
> There was only one set of footprints.
> I realized that this was at the lowest
> and saddest times of my life.
> This always bothered me
> and I questioned the Lord
> about my dilemma.

'Lord, you told me when I decided
to follow You,
You would walk and talk with me
all the way.
But I'm aware that during the most
troublesome times of my life
there is only one set of footprints.
I just don't understand why,
when I needed You most,
You leave me.'
He whispered, 'My precious child,
I love you and will never leave you
never, ever, during your trials and
testings.
When you saw only one set of footprints
it was then that I carried you.'

(Copyright © 1964 by Margaret Fishback Powers.)

The author has recently undertaken studies in psychology and professional counselling and is now a practising professional counsellor. If you would like to contact the author, write to:

PO Box 106
Williamstown VIC 3016.

Support groups and other resources

Support, self-help groups and carer associations

ACT

Canberra Manic-depressive Support Group
Pat Daniels
28 Paloona Place
Duffy ACT 2611
(062) 88 2747

Carers Association Inc.
(008) 817 746
Reply Paid 69 Woden
GPO Box 9832
Canberra ACT 2601
(to obtain copy of kit titled 'Carer Support: Practical Information on Caring at Home')

New South Wales

ARAFMI
PO Box 302
Cox Road
North Ryde NSW 2113
(02) 887 5766

Depressive and Manic Depressive Association of NSW
Subscriptions and enquiries:
DMDA Subscriptions
41 Ilka Street
Lilyfield NSW 2040
(details of support groups in and around the Sydney area are available by writing to this address)

Mental Health Information Service
9 a.m. – 5 p.m. weekdays
(02) 816 5688
For information on counselling, support groups, hospitals, accommodation, legal matters, telephone support, crisis services, family and other matters.

Northern Beaches Manic-depressive Self-help Group
Iris Hardcastle
Dee Why Community Health Centre
17 Pacific Parade
Dee Why NSW 2099
(02) 982 9155

MANDA Newcastle Organisation
Robyn Sanderson,
PO Box 2017,
Dangar NSW 2309
(049) 51 3589

Hunter Institute of Mental Health
72 Watt Street,
(PO Box 833),
Newcastle 2300
(049) 25 7813

GROW
Sydney NSW 2000
(02) 569 5566

CARE
Counselling & retraining for employment
6 Brighton Street
Croydon NSW 2132
(02) 747 5311 (ext 329) or 747 6289

Carers Association Inc.
(008) 817 023,
Reply Paid 69 Woden
GPO Box 9832
Sydney 2001
(to obtain copy of kit titled 'Carer Support: Practical Information on Caring at Home')

Queensland
Brisbane Manic-depressive Support Group
Friendship House
20 Balfour Street
New Farm QLD 4005
(07) 3358 4988

Ipswich Manic-depressive Support Group
John Hildebrand
Ipswich QLD 4305
(07) 3282 3781

Moodswing Illness Prevention
Suzanne Wootton
c/- Townsville Women's Centre
50 Patrick Street
Aitkenvale QLD 4814
(077) 75 7555

GROW
Brisbane QLD
(07) 3394 4344

Carers Association Inc.
(008) 017 223
Reply Paid 69 Woden
GPO Box 9832
Brisbane QLD 4001
(to obtain copy of kit titled 'Carer Support: Practical Information on Caring at Home')

South Australia
Edwards Crossing Community House
Hazel Pobke
18 Beatie Terrace
Murray Bridge SA 5253
(085) 32 6088

South Australia Self Help (MDP)
PO Box 153
Eastwood SA 5063
(08) 373 0088

GROW
Adelaide SA
(08) 297 6933

Carers Association Inc.
(008) 815 549
GPO Box 9832
Adelaide SA 5001
(to obtain copy of kit titled 'Carer Support: Practical Information on Caring at Home')

Victoria
ARAFEMI (Association of Relatives & Friends of the Emotionally and Mentally Ill)
615 Camberwell Road
Camberwell VIC 3124
(03) 9889 3733
Support Line: (03) 9889 1777 (available until 9 p.m.)
ARAFEMI can provide information about various Mutual Support Groups and Relatives and Friends Support Groups which operate in Melbourne metropolitan and some country areas.

Geelong Bipolar Disorder Support Group Inc.
June Plate
Barwon Psychiatric Resources Council
Ryrie Street

Geelong VIC 3220
(052) 29 8295
(052) 21 8722

GROW
29 Erasmus Street
Surrey Hills VIC 3127
(03) 9890 9846

Wodonga Psychiatric Rehabilitation Service
107 Hume Street
Wodonga VIC 3690
(060) 561700

EPPIC Centre
35 Poplar Road
Parkville VIC 3052
(03) 9389 2403
(videos and pamphlets available as well as inpatient and outpatient care)

Anorexia & Bulimia Nervosa Foundation of Victoria
1513 High Street
Glen Iris VIC 3146
(03) 9885 0318
(mood swings are a symptom of both illnesses, depression itself can be a
contributing factor)

Pathway Centre (children and adolescents 11 yrs to 21 yrs catered for)
24 Mercer Road
Armadale VIC 3143
(03) 9822 4644

Carers Association Victoria Inc.
(008) 9814 215
GPO Box 9832
Melbourne VIC 3001
(to obtain copy of kit titled 'Carer Support: Practical Information on
Caring at Home')

Western Australia

Wish Foundation
(Western Institute of Self Help)
80 Railway Street
Cottesloe WA 6011
(09) 383 3188
(008) 195 575
The Wish Foundation can provide information about the various Mutual
Support Groups which are operating in and around Perth.

Even Keel Manic-depressive Support Association Inc.
PO Box 1584
Midland WA 6056
Office: Tuesday 9.30 a.m. to 12.30 p.m.
(09) 274 2848 – Meetings at Mirrabooka, Fremantle and Midland

MIND
PO Box 1338
Midland WA 6056
(09) 255 1006

ARAFMI
(includes Young ARAFMI for young people)
2 Nicholson Road
Subiaco WA 6008
(09) 381 4747

ARAFMI
Esperance WA 6450
(090) 71 2566

ARAFMI
Geraldton WA 6530
(099) 21 2257
(099) 21 7833

ARAFMI
Central Wheatbelt WA
(096) 22 9583

WA Carers' Network Inc.
77 North Street
Mt Lawley WA 6050
(09) 272 2133

Carers Association Inc.
(008) 816 040
GPO Box 9832
Perth WA 6001
(to obtain copy of kit titled 'Carer Support: Practical Information on Caring at Home')

GROW
142 Beauford Street
PERTH 6000
(09) 328 3344

Tasmania
ARAFEMI
Hobart TAS 7000
(002) 24 1933

ARAFEMI
34 Howick Street
Launceston TAS 7250
(003) 27 3046

GROW
Hobart TAS 7000
(002) 23 6284

Carers Association Inc.
(008) 818 776
GPO Box 9832
Hobart TAS 7001

Tasmanian Association for Mental Health
PO Box 235
North Hobart TAS 7100
(002) 78 1608

Northern Territory
ARAFEMI
GPO Box 1370
Darwin NT 0801
(W) (08) 8981 4128

GROW
Drop-in Centre
Ground Floor
Casuarina Plaza
Casuarina NT 0810
(08) 8945 4096

Carers Association Inc.
Northern Territory
(008) 817 901

New Zealand
Otago Manic Depressive Support Trust Community Health Services
154 Hanover Street
Dunedin NZ
(Barbara and Jenny)
4740-999 (ext 7033)

Mental Health Foundation of New Zealand
PO Box 10051
Auckland NZ 1103
(09) 630 8573

Help with fears, phobias ...

Ansett Australia
Fear of Flying Program
Melbourne (03) 9339 5155
Sydney (02) 693 8323
Brisbane (07) 3867 2106
Adelaide (08) 238 1255
Perth (09) 334 1557

Western Australia
Agoraphobic Support
c/- Living Stone Foundation
2 Thorogood Street
Victoria Park WA 6100
(09) 470 4299
(telephone support, counselling, referral)

Northern Territory
Eating Disorders Self-help Group
Contact: 'Lani'
(Darwin)
(W) (08) 8982 1236
(H) (08) 8948 0472

Victoria
Anorexia & Bulimia Nervosa Foundation of Victoria (Inc)
1513 High Street
Glen Iris VIC 3146
(03) 9885 0318

Victorian Agoraphobia Centres
Box Hill	9890 2220
Laverton	9369 2022
Melton	9743 2022
Toorak	9347 7426
	9579 0007
Watsonia	9435 9777
Doveton/Hallam	9435 9777

Victorian Country Agoraphobia Centres

Shepparton   (058) 214 161
Mildura   (050) 236 342

Help for drug dependency

Victoria

Australian Drug Foundation
PO Box 529
South Melbourne VIC 3205
(03) 9416 1818
(outside Melbourne: 008 136 385)

TRANX Inc. Pty Ltd
(Tranquilliser Recovery and New Existence Inc.)
2 Rutland Road
Box Hill VIC 3128
(03) 9899 6078, 9899 6079
(counselling, telephone counselling Australia-wide, advisory service, support groups, networking, medical back-up, other resources)

Evancourt Private Hospital
(Recovery Centre for Alcohol & Minor Tranquilliser Dependencies and Stress Related Disorders)
1017 Dandenong Road
East Malvern VIC 3145
(03) 9571 5111 (toll-free: 008 809 600)
(many support groups meet at Evancourt such as Rational Recovery, Drug Independency, Alanon, Family Information Group, Womens Support Group, AA)

Westadd Inc.
49 Nicholson Street
Footscray VIC 3011
(03) 9689 5533

New South Wales
Australian Drug Foundation
(02) 331 2111
(outside Sydney: 008 422 599)

Queensland
Australian Drug Foundation
(07) 236 2414
(outside Brisbane: 008 177 833)

South Australia
Australian Drug Foundation
(08) 13 1340

Western Australia
Australian Drug Foundation
(09) 421 1900
(outside Perth: 008 198 024)

Tasmania
Australian Drug Foundation
(002) 288 220

ACT
Australian Drug Foundation
(06) 205 4545

Northern Territory
Australian Drug Foundation
(08) 8981 8030
(08) 8981 7516

ADF Information Line
0055 222 99

Mental Health Associations

ACT
Mental Health Foundation (ACT)
Level 5 Tower Building
Acton ACT 2601
(06) 247 5861

New South Wales
NSW Association for Mental Health
63 Victoria Road
Gladesville NSW 2111
(02) 816 1611

Victoria
Australian National Association for Mental Health
Tweedie Place
Richmond VIC 3121
(03) 9427 0373

Mental Health Foundation (Victoria)
Tweedie Place
Richmond VIC 3121
(03) 9427 0373

South Australia
Mental Health Association & Resource Centre (SA) Inc.
35 Fullarton Road
Kent Town SA 5067
(08) 362 6772

Queensland
Qld Association for Mental Health
Friendship House
20 Balfour Street
New Farm QLD 4005
(07) 358 4988

Northern Territory
NT Association for Mental Health
GPO Box 1370
Darwin NT 0801
(08) 8981 4128

Tasmania
Tas Association for Mental Health
PO Box 235
North Hobart TAS 7100
(002) 78 1557

Western Australia
WA Association for Mental Health
2 Nicholson Street
Subiaco WA 6008
(09) 381 1986

New Zealand
Mental Health Foundation of New Zealand
PO Box 10051
Auckland NZ 1103
(09) 630 8573

References and suggested reading

Aisbett, Bev, *Living with IT, A Survivor's Guide to Panic Attacks,* Angus & Robertson, Sydney, 1994.

American Psychiatric Association, *Diagnostic and Statistical Manual of Mental Disorders*, 3rd edn, American Psychiatric Association, Washington, 1980: 225–39.

Appleby, Margaret & Condonis, Margaret, *Hearing the Cry – Suicide Prevention*, ROSE Education Training & Consultancy, Narellan, NSW.

ARAFEMI Victoria, Australia, 'The Experience of Caregiving, Family Carers and Their Needs, Children of Parents Experiencing Major Mental Illness', Newsletter no. 51, September 1993.

Barnett, Dr Bryanne, *Coping With Postnatal Depression,* Lothian, Melbourne.

Brockington, I. F. & Kumar, R. (eds), *Motherhood and Mental Illness,* Academic Press, London, 1982.

Burns, David, *The Feeling Good Handbook,* William Morrow, New York, 1989.

Calabrese, J. R. & Delucchi, G. A., 'Spectrum of Efficacy of Valproate in 55 Patients with Rapid-cycling Bipolar Disorder', *American Journal of Psychiatry,* 1990; 147:431.

Coryell W., Noyes R. & Clancy J., 'Excess Mortality in Panic Disorder: A Comparison with Primary Unipolar Depression', *Archives of General Psychiatry*, 1982; 39:736–42.

Crowe R. R., Noyes R., Pauls D. L. & Slymen D. A., 'Family Study of Panic Disorder', *Archives of General Psychiatry,* 1983; 40:1968–9.

Duke, Patty & Hochman, Gloria, *A Brilliant Madness*, Bantam Books, New York, 1992.

Fieve, Dr Ronald R., *Moodswings*, Bantam Books, London, 1976.

Frampton, Muriel, *Agoraphobia: Coming to Terms with the World Outside,* Thorsons, England, 1990.

Frank, A.F. & Gunderson, J.G., 'The role of the therapeutic alliance in the treatment of schizophrenia: Relationship to course and outcome', *Archives and General Psychiatry*, 1990; 47:228–36.

Gillett, Richard, *Overcoming Depression, A Practical Self-help Guide to Prevention and Treatment,* Dorling Kindersley, London, 1987; Lothian, Melbourne, 1988.

Grounds, David & Armstrong, June, *Ecstasy & Agony,* Lothian, Melbourne, 1992.

Hales, Dianne, 'Depression', *The Encyclopedia of Health*, Chelsea House, Philadelphia, 1989.

Hatfield, Agnes B. & Lefley, Harriet P., *Families of the Mentally Ill*, The Guilford Press, USA, 1987.

Hoehn-Saric R., 'Neurotransmitters in Anxiety', *Archives of General Psychiatry*, 1982; 39:736–42.

Huszonek, J. J., 'Establishing therapeutic contact with schizophrenics: A supervisory approach', *American Journal of Psychotherapy*, 1987; 41:185–93.

Hyde, Margaret O. & Forsyth, Elizabeth H., *Suicide: The Hidden Epidemic,* Franklin Watts, New York, London, 1978.

Judd, Fiona K. & Burrows, Graham D., 'Panic and Phobic Disorders', *Australian Family Physician*, vol. 15, no. 2, February 1986.

Kaplan, H. I. and Sadock, B. J. (eds), *Comprehensive Text Book of Psychiatry*, 5th edn, vol. 1, 1989.

Katon, W. 'Panic Disorder and Somatisation', *Am J. Med*, 1984; 77:101–6.

Kuipers, Liz & Bebbington, Paul, *Living with Mental Illness*, Souvenir Press (Educational & Academic), London, 1987.

Kulkarni, Jayashri & Singh, Bruce, 'Mood Disorders and Anticonvulsants', *Australian Prescriber*, vol. 15, no. 1, 1992.

Kumar, R. & Brockington, I. (eds), *Motherhood and Mental Illness 2 – Causes and Consequences,* Wright, London, 1988.

Lewis, David, *Fight Your Phobia – and Win,* Sheldon Press, London, 1984.

McGorry, Patrick D., 'The Concept of Recovery and Secondary Prevention in Psychotic Disorders', *Australian and New Zealand Journal of Psychiatry,* 1992; 26:3–17.

McGorry, Patrick D., 'Early Psychosis Prevention and Intervention Centre', *Australasian Psychiatry*, vol. 1, no. 1, April 1993.

McKinnon, Pauline, *In Stillness Conquer Fear,* Dove Communications, Melbourne, 1983.

McLellan, Betty. *Overcoming Anxiety, A Positive Approach to Dealing With Severe Anxiety in Your Life,* Allen & Unwin, Sydney, 1992.

Maltz, Maxwell, *The Magic Power of Self-Image Psychology*, Pocket Books (Simon & Schuster), New York, 1970.

Maltz, Maxwell, *Psycho-Cybernetics,* Pocket Books (Simon & Schuster), New York, 1969.

Matthews A. M., Teasdale J., Munby M., Johnston D. & Shaw P., 'A Home Based Treatment Programme for Agoraphobia', *Behav Ther,* 1977; 8:915–24.

Miles, Robert, *Conquer Fear of Flying,* Millennium Books, Newtown NSW, 1993, self-published Melbourne, 1993.

Milligan, Spike & Clare, Anthony, *Depression and How to Survive It,* Edbury Press, London, 1993.

Mitchell, Phillip, 'Anticonvulsants Use in Mood Disorders', *Current Therapeutics*, February 1992.

Mitchell, Phillip, 'Psychiatry', *Australian Prescriber*, vol. 14, no. 3, 1991.

Montgomery, Bob, *The Truth about Success and Motivation,* Lothian, Melbourne, 1987.

Montgomery, Bob & Morris, Laurel, *Living With Anxiety,* Lothian, Melbourne, 1992.

National Depressive and Manic-Depressive Association, Chicago, *In Bipolar Illness: Rapid Cycling & Its Treatment,* undated brochure.

National Depressive and Manic-Depressive Association, Chicago, *When Treatments Fail, Depression & Manic Depression,* undated brochure.

Neuman, Frederic, *Fighting Fear,* Macmillan, New York, 1985.

Noyes R., Clancy J., Hoenk P. R. & Slymer D. J., 'Anxiety Neurosis and Physical Illness, *Compr Psychiatry*, 1978; 19: 407–13.

Okuma T et al. 'Anti-manic Prophylactic Effects of Carbamazepine (Tegretol) on Manic-depressive Psychosis: A Preliminary Report', *Folia Psychiatry and Neurology*, 1973; 27:283–97.

Papolos, Dimitri & Janice, *Overcoming Depression,* Harper & Row, New York, 1988.

Priest, Robert, *Anxiety and Depression, A Practical Guide to Recovery*, Macdonald Optima, London, 1988.

Quitkin F. M., Rifkin A., Kaplan J., Klein D. F. & Oakes G., 'Phobic Anxiety Syndrome Complicated by Drug Dependence and Addiction', *Archives of General Psychiatry*, 1972; 27:159–62.

Robins L. N., Helzer J. E., Weissman M. M. et al., 'Lifetime Prevalence of Specific Psychiatric Disorders in Three Sites', *Archives of General Psychiatry*, 1984; 41:949–58.

Rossmanith, Angela, *The Self Alone: Understanding Loneliness in Our Lives*, Collins Dove, Melbourne, 1995.

Sanderson, Mikela, *Coping Strategies for Depression*, unpublished.

Schou, Mogens, *Lithium Treatment of Manic-Depressive Illness, A Practical Guide*, English Edition by S. Karger AG, Basel, Switzerland, 1989.

Sheehan, D. V., 'Panic Attacks and Phobias', *New England Journal of Medicine*, 1982; 307:156–8.

Styron, William, *Darkness Visible*, Jonathan Cape, London, 1991.

Tagore, R., quoted in *Noon to Nightfall*, M. D'Apice, Collins Dove, Melbourne, 1989.

Tranquilliser Recovery and New Existence (TRANX), *What To Do When You Reach the Bottom? Information for people taking sleeping pills and anti-anxiety tablets* and other TRANX brochures, Melbourne, undated.

Upfal, Jonathan, *The Australian Drug Guide*, Bookman Press, Melbourne, 1992.

Weekes, Claire, *Self Help for Your Nerves*, Angus & Robertson, Sydney, 1969, 1981.

Weekes, Claire, *Peace from Nervous Suffering,* Angus & Robertson, Sydney, 1981.

Weekes, Claire, *Simple Effective Treatment of Agoraphobia,* Angus & Robertson, Sydney, 1977.

Whitehead, Tony, *Overcoming Fears and Phobias,* Sheldon Press, London, 1980, 1988.